Second Edition

Clinical Primer
A POCKET GUIDE FOR DENTAL ASSISTANTS

Melanie Mitchell, CDA-Emeritus, BGS

Total Care Programming, Inc.

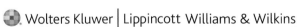 Wolters Kluwer | Lippincott Williams & Wilkins
Health
Philadelphia · Baltimore · New York · London
Buenos Aires · Hong Kong · Sydney · Tokyo

Acquisitions Editor: Chris Johnson
Product Manager: Paula C. Williams
Marketing Manager: Shauna Kelley

Designer: Holly McLaughlin
Compositor: Integra Software Services Pvt. Ltd.,
Vendor Manager: Alicia Jackson

Second Edition

Library of Congress Cataloging-in-Publication Data

Mitchell, Melanie, 1953–
    Clinical primer : a pocket guide for dental assistants / Melanie Mitchell. — 2nd ed.
      p. ; cm.
    Pocket guide for dental assistants
    ISBN 978-1-4511-0508-7 — ISBN 1-4511-0508-8
    I. Title.   II. Title: Pocket guide for dental assistants.
    [DNLM: 1. Dental Assistants—Handbooks.   2. Dentistry—methods—Handbooks. WU 49]

    617.6′0233—dc23

RRS1207

2012007463

DISCLAIMER

Care has been taken to confirm the accuracy of the information present and to describe generally accepted practices. However, the authors, editors, and publisher are not responsible for errors or omissions or for any consequences from application of the information in this book and make no warranty, expressed or implied, with respect to the currency, completeness, or accuracy of the contents of the publication. Application of this information in a particular situation remains the professional responsibility of the practitioner; the clinical treatments described and recommended may not be considered absolute and universal recommendations.

The authors, editors, and publisher have exerted every effort to ensure that drug selection and dosage set forth in this text are in accordance with the current recommendations and practice at the time of publication. However, in view of ongoing research, changes in government regulations, and the constant flow of information relating to drug therapy and drug reactions, the reader is urged to check the package insert for each drug for any change in indications and dosage and for added warnings and precautions. This is particularly important when the recommended agent is a new or infrequently employed drug.

Some drugs and medical devices presented in this publication have Food and Drug Administration (FDA) clearance for limited use in restricted research settings. It is the responsibility of the health care provider to ascertain the FDA status of each drug or device planned for use in their clinical practice.

To purchase additional copies of this book, call our customer service department at (800) 638-3030 or fax orders to (301) 223-2320. International customers should call (301) 223-2300.

Visit Lippincott Williams & Wilkins on the Internet: http://www.lww.com. Lippincott Williams & Wilkins customer service representatives are available from 8:30 am to 6:00 pm, EST.

About the Author

Melanie Mitchell was employed as a clinical dental assistant in orthodontics and general practice before becoming an instructor and director of the Dental Assistant Program at the Wichita Area Technical College (WATC). Melanie recently retired after 25 years as the director of the Dental Assistant Program and continues to serve as an adjunct instructor at WATC. She has been a DANB Certified Dental Assistant since 1972. She is a life member of the American Dental Assistants Association and has held numerous leadership positions at both the local level and state level. Melanie received the American Dental Assistant Association Sullivan-Schein Award of Excellence in 1999. She has also written ***Dental Instruments: A Pocket Guide to Identification***.

Reviewers

Julie Bera, CDA, COA, RDA, MA
Professor
Grand Rapids Community College
Grand Rapids, Michigan

Sharron J. Cook, CDA
Program Director/Instructor, Dental Assisting
Columbus Technical College,
Columbus, Georgia

Carol Anne Giaquinto, CDA, RDH, M.Ed.
Program Coordinator, Dental Assisting
Springfield Technical Community College
Springfield, Massachusetts

Kay Hudak, CDA, CDPMA
Instructor, Dental Assisting
Lancaster County Career and Technology Center
Willow Street, Pennsylvania

Donna Schultz Lepkoski, CDA, EFDA, FADAA, BS
Professor, Dental Health Programs
Luzerne County Community College
Nanticoke, Pennsylvania

Martha McCaslin, CDA, MA
Program Director, Dental Assisting
Dona Ana Community College
Las Cruces, New Mexico

Vicky Parrott, CDA, RDA
Program Director, Dental Assisting
Vatterott College
Springfield, Missouri

Le Ann Schoenle, LDA, CDA, RF, BS
Program Director, Dental Assisting
Central Lakes College
Brainerd, Minnesota

Angela E. Simmons, CDA, CPFDA, BS
Dental Assisting Department Chair
Fayetteville Technical Community College
Fayetteville, North Carolina

Deborah J. Smith, CDA, BS
Program Coordinator/ Dental Assistant
Milwaukee Area Technical College
Milwaukee, Wisconsin

Diana M. Sullivan, MS, CDA, LDA
Program Director
Dakota County Technical College
Rosemont, Minnesota

Cynthia Phillips-Wood, RDA
Program Chair, Dental Assisting
Anthem College/HT
Irving, Texas

Preface

Clinical Primer: A Pocket Guide for Dental Assistants is written as a resource for review of the core knowledge and skills needed in clinical dental practice. This textbook is a useful reference book for students in the transition from classroom to clinical practice and also for employees new to dentistry. It is designed as a pocket reference that can be taken with the learner into the clinical setting.

The ***Clinical Primer*** is written in a concise, practical manner using diagrams, photos, tables, charts, bulleted lists, procedural tray setups, and step-by-step clinical procedures. The Student Resources on CD-ROM packaged with this text and online on thePoint, www.thepoint.lww.com/mitchellclinical2e, deliver expanded dental material information with web links, photos of tray set ups and instruments, charting, procedure video clips, reference materials, and activities to reinforce learning.

This 2nd edition of the ***Clinical Primer*** includes new chapters on assessing patient vital signs and on dental health and prevention information to enhance patient education skills. The 2nd edition has also been expanded with additional step-by-step clinical procedures and expanded functions, updated photos and diagrams, and additional tray setups.

Acknowledgments

James Booth, Instructional Design and Programming
Kathryn Booth, Instructional Design
Karen Callanan, D.D.S., Consultant
Christopher Johnson, Acquisitions Editior/Publisher, Lippincott Williams & Wilkins
Paula Williams, Product Manager, Lippincott Williams & Wilkins
Holly McLaughlin, Design Coordinator, Lippincott Williams & Wilkins
Alicia Jackson, Vendor Manager, Lippincott Williams & Wilkins

A special thanks to my family for their patience, loving support, and encouragement.

Contents

Photo and Illustration Credits

Tooth Anatomy, Eruption Dates, and Numbering Systems

Coronal Anatomy—Number and Location of Cusps on Permanent Premolars and Molars

TABLE 1-1 Number and Location of Cusps on Permanent Premolars and Molars

	Number of cusps	Location of cusps
Maxillary 1st and 2nd premolars	2	Buccal and lingual
Mandibular 1st premolar	2	Buccal and lingual
Mandibular 2nd premolar	Often 3	Buccal, mesiolingual, and distolingual
Maxillary 1st molar	5	Mesiobuccal, distobuccal, mesiolingual, distolingual, and cusp of Carabelli (on lingual of mesiolingual cusp)
Maxillary 2nd molar	4	Mesiobuccal, distobuccal, mesiolingual, and distolingual
Mandibular 1st molar	5	Mesiobuccal, distobuccal, distal (smallest), mesiolingual, and distolingual
Mandibular 2nd molar	4	Mesiobuccal, distobuccal, mesiolingual, and distolingual

Roots and Pulp Canals

All anterior teeth, the maxillary 2nd premolar, and the mandibular 1st and 2nd premolars generally have one root and one canal. Multirooted teeth are identified in Table 1-2.

TABLE 1-2 Multirooted Permanent Teeth

	Number and location of roots	Number and location of canals
Maxillary 1st premolar	2 roots—buccal and lingual	2 canals—buccal and lingual
Maxillary 1st and 2nd molars	3 roots—mesiobuccal, distobuccal, and lingual	3 canals—mesiobuccal, distobuccal, and lingual
Mandibular 1st and 2nd molars	2 roots—mesial and distal	3 canals—mesiobuccal, mesiolingual, and distal

TOOTH ID 1

Eruption Dates—Primary and Permanent Teeth

TABLE 1-3 Primary Dentition Eruption Dates

Primary teeth	Eruption date	Exfoliation date
Central incisors	6–8 months	6–7 years
Lateral incisors	8–10 months	7–8 years
Canines	16–20 months	9–12 years
1st molars	12–16 months	9–11 years
2nd molars	20–30 months	9–11 years

TABLE 1-4 Permanent Dentition Eruption Dates

Permanent teeth	Eruption date
Central incisors	6–7 years (mandibular), 7–8 years (maxillary)
Lateral incisors	8–9 years
Canines	11–12 years
1st premolars	10–11 years
2nd premolars	10–12 years
1st molars	6–7 years
2nd molars	12–13 years
3rd molars	17–21 years

In the universal numbering system, each permanent tooth has a unique number and each primary tooth has a unique letter as shown in Figure 1-1.

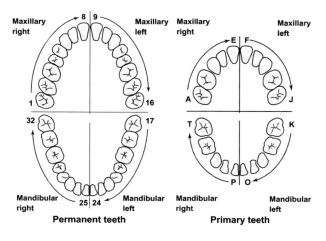

Permanent teeth

Primary teeth

Tooth Numbering—Palmer's System

In the Palmer's numbering system, the tooth number (permanent) or the tooth letter (primary) is combined with the quadrant symbol (shown in green, Figure 1-2) to create a unique identifier for each tooth. For example, the maxillary left permanent 1st molar is denoted as $\underline{6}$ and the mandibular right primary 1st molar is denoted as $\overline{\mathrm{d}}$.

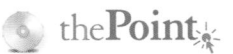 the**Point**

CD-ROM includes review for this chapter.

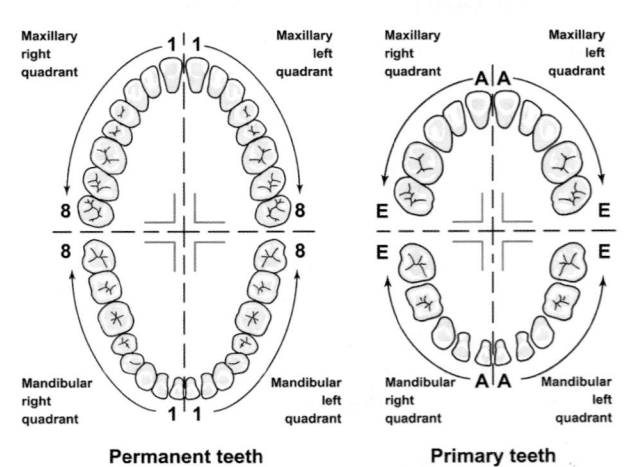

Permanent teeth   **Primary teeth**

Dental Health and Prevention

Dental Decay—Conversation Points for Patient Education

Dental decay is caused by bacteria normally present in the mouth. When the bacteria combine with the sugars and starches in food, acid is created that dissolves minerals in the tooth surface (this process is called decalcification or demineralization). With repeated acid attacks, a cavity can form. In summary,

Bacteria + sugar = acid

Acid + tooth surface = decay

A clear film known as the acquired pellicle forms on tooth surfaces within minutes after brushing the teeth. This film provides a surface onto which bacteria can easily attach and rapidly multiply. This is the first stage in plaque formation. Plaque is a soft, sticky bacterial film that must be removed daily to prevent dental disease.

Plaque that remains on tooth surfaces for more than 24 hours can cause disease.

In addition, minerals in saliva combine with plaque to form a rough, hard deposit known as calculus. These hard deposits irritate the gum tissues and prevent effective home care. Calculus cannot be removed with regular brushing and flossing.

Decay is most likely to occur in grooves and pits and also on smooth surfaces where removing plaque is difficult.

Preventing Decay

- Brush teeth twice daily with fluoride toothpaste
- Use a soft bristled toothbrush and replace it every 3 to 4 months
- Floss daily to clean adjacent tooth surfaces
- Avoid between-meal snacks and eat a balanced diet
- Visit a dentist regularly for teeth cleaning and oral examination

Periodontal tissues include the *gingiva, alveolar bone, periodontal ligament*, and *cementum* (Figure 2-1).

Periodontal disease is caused by bacteria normally present in the mouth. The inflammatory response to the irritants produced by the bacteria has an effect on the progression of periodontal disease.

The bacteria in dental plaque produce toxins that irritate the gingiva and cause gingival inflammation known as *gingivitis*. Clinical signs include gingival redness, swelling, and bleeding.

Background Information: A clear film known as the acquired pellicle forms on tooth surfaces within minutes after brushing the teeth. This film provides a surface onto which bacteria can easily attach and rapidly multiply. This is the first stage in the formation of a soft, sticky bacterial film known as plaque. Plaque must be removed daily to prevent dental disease.

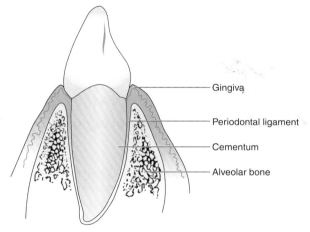

Gingiva
Periodontal ligament
Cementum
Alveolar bone

FIGURE 2–1 Cross-sectional view of the supporting tissues of the teeth.

9

Dental
Health
2

In addition, minerals in saliva combine with plaque to form a rough, hard deposit known as calculus. These hard deposits irritate the gingiva and prevent effective home care. Calculus cannot be removed with regular brushing and flossing.

Gingivitis can be eliminated with professional treatment and good oral hygiene.

If plaque and calculus are not removed, gingival inflammation can continue into the deeper periodontal tissues—bone, periodontal ligament, and cementum. Inflammation of these deeper tissues is known as *periodontitis*.

Tissue Changes and Clinical Signs Associated with Periodontitis

- Rolled, rounded, blunted, or cratered gingiva
- Gingival recession
- Pus
- Periodontal pockets
- Radiographic bone loss
- Tooth mobility

Gingival recession and bone loss from periodontitis can be controlled. With treatment, the progression of the disease can be stopped and tissues can be restored to a healthy state.

Preventing Periodontal Disease

- Brush teeth twice daily with fluoride toothpaste
- Use a soft bristled toothbrush and replace it every 3 to 4 months
- Floss daily to clean adjacent tooth surfaces
- Avoid between-meal snacks and eat a balanced diet
- Visit a dentist regularly for teeth cleaning and oral examination

Factors That Increase the Risk of Developing Periodontal Disease

- Tobacco use
- Hormonal changes
- Systemic diseases such as diabetes
- Badly positioned teeth
- Poor bite relationship
- Medications such as steroids, some antiepilepsy drugs and oral contraceptives, and cancer therapy drugs

Dental Health 2

Providing Brushing Instructions—Bass Technique

Brushing removes plaque from the facial, lingual, and occlusal surfaces of the teeth.

There are a number of toothbrushing techniques. The Bass technique is the one most commonly used for older children and adults.

Equipment Needed: Dental Manikin and Toothbrushes in a Variety of Designs and Sizes

Step-by-Step Procedure

1. Explain the relationship of plaque to dental disease.
2. Discuss where plaque is located, the importance of removing plaque, and the recommended frequency of removing plaque.
3. Advise patient that a soft bristled toothbrush is best for the soft tissues and more easily conforms to the contours of the teeth. The toothbrush should be replaced every 3 months.
4. Demonstrate the Bass technique on the manikin beginning with the facial of the maxillary molars:
   - Place the toothbrush near the gingival margin at a 45° angle to the root of the tooth (Figure 2-2). Using light pressure, vibrate the bristles back and forth without dislodging the bristle tips, then stroke the bristles toward the occlusal.

- Move the brush forward, a little less than the full length of the brush, and repeat the process around the maxillary arch.
- Repeat the procedure for the facial of the mandibular teeth.
- Use the same technique for the lingual surfaces of both maxillary and mandibular posterior teeth.
- To clean the lingual surfaces of the anterior teeth, place the head of the toothbrush vertically, gently move the brush back and forth, then stroke the bristles toward the incisal (Figure 2-3).
- On all occlusal surfaces, hold the bristles flat against the surface and brush back and forth or in a circular motion.
- Also brush the tongue in a back-to-front sweeping motion to remove bacteria and food particles.

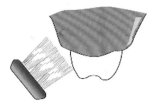

FIGURE 2–2 Toothbrush near the gingival margin at a 45° angle.

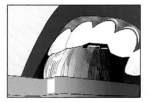

FIGURE 2–3 Toothbrush placement for lingual surfaces of the anterior teeth.

5. Encourage the patient to ask questions and watch for nonverbal signs of understanding.
6. Ask the patient to demonstrate the technique to verify understanding.

Providing Flossing Instructions

Equipment Needed: Dental Manikin and Dental Floss

Step-by-Step Procedure
1. Explain that plaque readily forms on the proximal surfaces of the teeth and is not removed by brushing.
2. Using a manikin, demonstrate flossing:
   - Wrap one end of the floss strip around the middle finger of the right hand. Next, wrap the length of the floss around the left middle finger, leaving 2" to 3" of working space (Figure 2-4).
   - Stretch the floss tightly between the fingers and using the thumbs or index fingers to guide the floss, ease the floss through the contact area with a gentle back and forth motion.
   - Curve the floss tightly around the proximal side of one tooth (Figure 2-5).
   - Move the floss down to the sulcus area and back up to the contact area, repeat several times.
   - Curve the floss tightly around the proximal side of the adjacent tooth.

- Move the floss down to the sulcus area and back up to the contact area, repeat several times.
- Repeat procedure on each tooth in both arches.
- Unwind a clean strip of floss after every two to three teeth.
- Always floss the distal surface of the most posterior tooth in each quadrant.

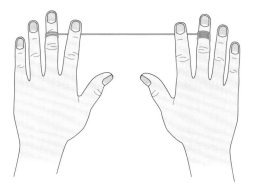

FIGURE 2–4 Floss wrapped around the middle fingers.

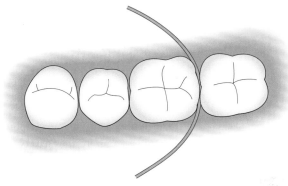

FIGURE 2–5 Floss curved tightly against the proximal surface.

3. Instruct the patient to avoid back and forth movements of the floss once the floss is through the contact area. The floss can cut the gingiva if not used correctly.

4. Inform the patient gingival bleeding or soreness may occur when first starting regular flossing. If bleeding continues beyond the first week, the patient should call the dental office.

5. Encourage the patient to ask questions and watch for nonverbal signs of understanding.

6. Ask the patient to demonstrate the technique to verify understanding.

Dental Health Information: Internet Resources

www.ada.org/public.aspx

www.perio.org

www.dentalcare.com

www.cdc.gov/oralhealth

http://ada.org/286.aspx

Daily Routine and Care of Treatment Area

Preparation at the Beginning of the Day

1. Report to the office 15 to 30 minutes before the first scheduled patient.
2. Change into clinical attire.
3. Switch on the air compressor, central vacuum unit, sterilizers, computers, darkroom safelights, and automatic processor.

4. Check daily schedule and review the first patient's chart.

5. Place current radiographs on viewbox.

6. Wash hands and put on a mask and gloves.

7. Switch on units in each treatment room.

8. If unit equipped with an independent water supply, fill water bottles and attach to unit (Figure 3-1).

9. Flush handpiece tubing (discharge water from tubing without handpiece attached) and air/water syringe for 30 to 60 seconds.

   Note: Discharging water from the lines at the beginning of each day removes the bacterial colonies that have formed in the waterlines overnight. Remember to flush into the suction tubing to reduce airborne microbes.

10. Discard the gloves and mask and wash hands.

11. Place plastic barriers on chair, unit, and light.

12. Select proper tray setup and materials for scheduled procedure.

13. After patient is seated, attach the sterile handpieces (high and low speed), air/water syringe tips, oral evacuator tip, and disposable saliva ejector tip as needed.

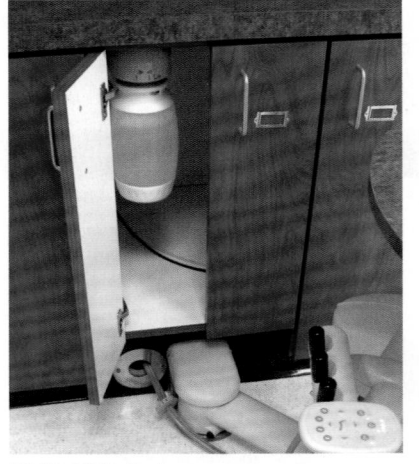

FIGURE 3–1 Dental unit water supply.

Decontaminate the Treatment Area after a Procedure

1. While wearing treatment gloves
   - run high-speed handpiece, with bur in place, over suction for 20 to 30 seconds;
   - remove evacuation tips, air/water syringe tips, and handpieces and place on instrument tray;
   - remove soiled barriers and place on instrument tray;
   - take instrument tray with contaminated items to contaminated area of sterilization room;
   - remove anesthetic needle and carpule from syringe and place in **sharps container**;
   - place any bloody waste in **biohazard** container and other waste in regular trash can;
   - place soiled instruments in ultrasonic basket (except for handpieces).
2. Remove treatment gloves, wash hands, and don clean utility gloves.
3. While wearing utility gloves
   - clean and disinfect tray (spray–wipe–spray) and towel clips and place in clean area;
   - return to treatment room and activate rheostat to flush handpiece waterline into suction tubing for 20 to 30 seconds;
   - apply cleaner/disinfectant to all non-barrier covered surfaces (counter tops, tubing and hoses, dental chair, control pads and switches, assistant and operator's stools);

19

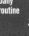

Daily routine

3

- ■ vigorously wipe all sprayed surfaces with 4×4 gauze or paper towels;
- ■ reapply disinfectant to all surfaces and leave wet for manufacturer's recommended time (3 to 10 minutes).
4. Wash utility gloves, dry, remove, and spray with disinfectant.
5. Remove mask and protective eyewear; wash hands.
6. Place new barriers.

Removing Contaminated Treatment Gloves

1. Remove contaminated gloves before removing other contaminated personal protective equipment (PPE—protective eyewear, mask, and gown).
2. Remove the first glove by pinching a portion of the glove near the wrist and palm. Pull out and away and slide the hand out of the glove (Figure 3-2).
3. Keep holding the soiled glove as you place the two fingers of your ungloved hand under the cuff of the second glove (Figure 3-3).
4. Pull the glove up and away toward the fingertips of the gloved hand as you turn the glove inside out with the first glove balled up inside it. Take care not to touch the outside of the glove.
5. Discard the contaminated gloves and wash your hands.

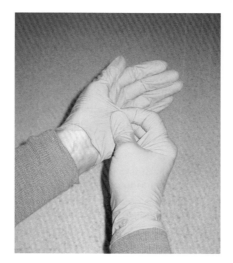

FIGURE 3–2 Removing contaminated gloves—step 1.

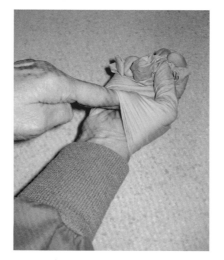

FIGURE 3–3 Removing contaminated gloves—step 2.

Daily routine

3

End-of-the-Day Routine

1. Complete steps to *decontaminate the treatment room after dental procedure (see previous page)*.

   In addition, while wearing utility gloves

   - activate rheostat to flush handpiece waterline into suction for 30 to 60 seconds;
   - check the saliva ejector trap and the unit's solid collection tank and empty or dispose of filters if debris present;
   - aspirate sanitizing solution through all suction hoses;
   - clean sinks in treatment room;
   - drain ultrasonic solution.

2. Wash utility gloves, dry, remove and disinfect; wash hands.
3. Restock consumable supplies.
4. If unit is equipped with independent water supply, remove and empty water bottle.
5. Turn off unit, sterilizers, central air compressor and vacuum unit, computers, darkroom safelights, and automatic processor.
6. Check the next day's appointment schedule to determine that all records have been compiled and any necessary lab work has been received.
7. Check that all lab cases have been sent to the lab or are ready to be sent.
8. Remove clinical attire and place in appropriate container.

Instrument Processing

1. Put on utility gloves, protective eyewear, and mask.
2. **Transport** contaminated instruments to processing area.
3. Place contaminated instruments in ultrasonic basket.
4. **Clean**—place cover on cleaning unit and process for manufacturer's recommended time: approximately 4 to 6 minutes for loose instruments and 10 to 16 minutes for cassettes.
5. Remove cover and lift out cleaning basket, rinse under tap water, and empty onto towel.
6. **Inspect** instruments for broken tips and cleanliness; replace or reclean as needed.
7. **Dry**—carefully pat with thick towel.
8. **Wrap/package** instruments in materials appropriate for selected sterilization process.
9. **Sterilize** instruments in an FDA-approved sterilizer—DO NOT OVERLOAD.
10. Use biological monitors weekly.
11. **Store** instruments in a clean, dry environment; rotate packages to use packages with oldest sterilization dates first.

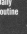

Daily
routine

3

High-Speed Handpiece Cleaning and Sterilization

While Wearing Appropriate PPE after Each Patient

1. Run handpiece, with bur in place, into suction for 20 to 30 seconds to flush bioburden from interior of handpiece and waterlines.
2. Disconnect handpiece from tubing.
3. In sterilization area, scrub external surface of handpiece with soap and water; dry.
4. Use automated handpiece maintenance device (Figure 3-4) OR place paper towel over head of instrument and spray pressurized cleaner/lubricant into the central tube in the back end of the handpiece until ejected solution comes out clean. Reattach handpiece to air/water system and flush out excess cleaner/lubricant.

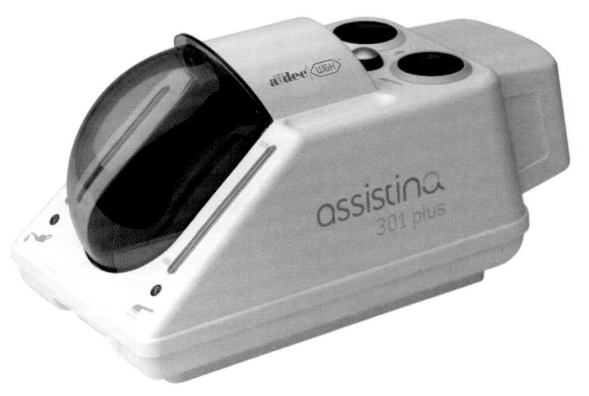

FIGURE 3-4 A-dec Assistina, automated handpiece maintenance device. Image courtesy of A-dec.

5. Wipe off any excess cleaner/lubricant from handpiece and place in sterilization bag.

6. Sterilize with steam heat sterilizer.

7. After sterilization cycle, when cool, open bag just enough to lubricate (if recommended by manufacturer).

Note: Recommended cleaning and sterilization procedures vary by manufacturer and by model of handpiece. Always *read and follow carefully* the manufacturer's specific instructions for cleaning, lubrication, and sterilization of handpieces.

Infection Control/Occupational Safety: Internet Resources

www.cdc.gov/mmwr

www.osha.gov

www.osap.org

Daily
routine
3

25

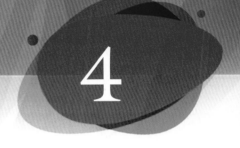

chapter

4

Patient Assessment

Measuring Blood Pressure

In adults, normal blood pressure is 120 mm Hg or less for systolic and 80 mm Hg or less for diastolic. Blood pressure is recorded as a fraction, for example, 120/80.

Equipment Needed

Sphygmomanometer (blood pressure cuff), stethoscope, and patient's chart.

Step-by-Step Procedure

1. Seat patient with back supported and legs uncrossed.
2. Extend patient's arm palm side up, place at heart level, and support on firm surface.
3. If necessary, push the patient's sleeve up to expose the upper arm.
4. Place the cuff around the patient's upper arm 1" above the antecubital space.
5. Place the bulb in your dominant hand and turn the valve screw to the right until it stops.
6. Palpate brachial artery (Figure 4-1).
7. Pump the bulb to inflate the cuff until you can no longer feel the brachial pulse and note the reading on the dial or mercury column.
8. Quickly turn the valve to the left (counterclockwise) to deflate the cuff completely. Wait for 30 seconds before reinflating the cuff.
9. Place the earpieces of the stethoscope, facing toward the eardrum, in your ears.

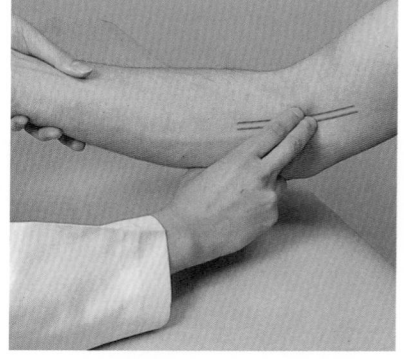

FIGURE 4–1 Locating the brachial artery. Reprinted with permission from Bickley LS, Szilagyi P. *Bates' Guide to Physical Examination and History Taking.* 8th ed. Philadelphia, PA: Lippincott Williams & Wilkins; 2003.

10. With your nondominant hand, place the diaphragm of the stethoscope on the brachial artery and hold firmly (Figure 4-2).

11. Turn the valve screw to close the valve and reinflate the cuff. Inflate to 30 mm Hg above the number at which the brachial artery was no longer felt.

12. Turn the valve screw counterclockwise at about 2 to 4 mm Hg per second.

13. Listen carefully and note the number at which the first sound is heard. This is the systolic measurement.

14. Continue listening and slowly deflating the cuff.

15. When you hear the last sound, note the reading and quickly deflate the cuff completely. The last sound is the diastolic measurement.

16. Remove the stethoscope from your ears. Remove the cuff from the patient's arm.

17. Record the blood pressure measurement in the patient's chart.

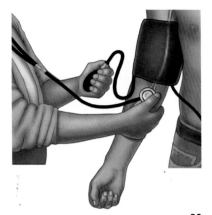

FIGURE 4–2 Measuring blood pressure. Reprinted with permission from McArdle WD, Katch FI, Katch VL. *Essentials of Exercise Physiology.* 2nd ed. Baltimore, MD: Lippincott Williams and Wilkins; 2000.

Patient
Assessment
4

Measuring Pulse Rate

Equipment Needed

Watch with a second hand and patient's chart.

TABLE 4-1	Pulse Rate by Age
Age (years)	**Normal pulse rate (beats per minute)**
3–6 (child)	75–120
6–12 (child)	75–110
>12 (adult)	60–100

Step-by-Step Procedure

1. Extend the patient's arm, supported on a firm surface.
2. Place the index and second finger gently but firmly on the radial artery located at the base of the thumb on the inside of the wrist (Figure 4-3).
3. Count the pulse for 30 seconds. Multiply that number by two to calculate beats per minute.
4. Record pulse rate in the patient's chart.

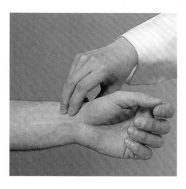

FIGURE 4–3 Locating the radial artery to measure pulse. Reprinted with permission from Bickley LS, Szilagyi P. *Bates' Guide to Physical Examination and History Taking.* 8th ed. Philadelphia, PA: Lippincott Williams & Wilkins; 2003.

Measuring Respirations

Patients may not breathe normally if they know that they are being assessed. Count respirations immediately before or after measuring the patient's pulse. Explain to the patient that you are taking their pulse; do not mention that you will also be measuring respiration rate.

31

Patient
Assessment
4

Equipment Needed

Watch with a second hand and patient's chart.

Step-by-Step Procedure

1. While the patient is in position for measuring pulse rate, watch the patient's chest/abdomen for breathing.
2. One respiration is the rise and fall of the patient's chest.
3. Count the respirations for 30 seconds. Multiply that number by two to calculate respiratory rate.
4. Record respiratory rate in the patient's chart.

TABLE 4–2 Respiration Rate by Age	
Age (years)	**Normal rate of respirations per minute**
3–6 (child)	20–30
6–12 (child)	18–25
>12 (adult)	12–20

TABLE 4–3 Basic Emergency Procedures

Emergency condition	Signs	Actions required
Syncope (fainting)	Pallor, sweating, loss of consciousness	Place patient in subsupine position. Administer ammonia inhalant. Monitor vital signs
Hyperventilation	Rapid breathing, faintness, numbness of extremities, nervousness	Remain calm. Assist patient in slowing breathing. Have patient breathe into bag or cupped hands
Epileptic seizures	Body jerking, twitching	Remove items from mouth and from area that could harm the patient. Do not restrain. Remain with patient

(Continued)

Patient
Assessment
4

TABLE 4-3 *(Continued)*

Emergency condition	Signs	Actions required
Heart attack	Chest discomfort, lasting more than 15–20 min, that is not relieved by rest and/or nitroglycerin. Other signs include sweating, nausea, weakness, and shortness of breath	Stop activity. Place patient in comfortable position. Call 911. Administer nitroglycerin and oxygen as determined by dentist. Monitor vital signs
Cardiac arrest	Loss of consciousness, breath, and pulse	Call 911. Begin CPR
Stroke	Sudden numbness or weakness of face, arm, or leg. Sudden confusion and trouble speaking or understanding. Sudden loss of balance or coordination. Sudden trouble seeing. Sudden severe headache with no known cause	Call 911

First Aid and Emergency Procedures: Internet Resources

www.mayoclinic.com/health/FirstAidIndex/FirstAidIndex

www.americanheart.org

chapter

5

Cavity Classifications and Dental Charting

Black's Cavity Classifications

Class I	All pit and fissure cavities
Class II	All proximal surface cavities of posterior teeth
Class III	Proximal surface cavities of anterior teeth that **do not** involve the incisal edge
Class IV	Proximal surface cavities of anterior teeth that **do** involve the incisal edge
Class V	All gingival 1/3 cavities
Class VI	Dentin exposure on incisal edge or occlusal surface (cusp tips) due to attrition

Dental Charting

Charting symbols are used to efficiently record existing conditions, treatment needed, and treatment performed.

Red symbols indicate treatment that needs to be performed and conditions that need attention. Blue symbols indicate treatment that has been performed previously (restorations, root canals, and sealants). Blue symbols also indicate existing conditions that do not require any treatment (for example, missing teeth).

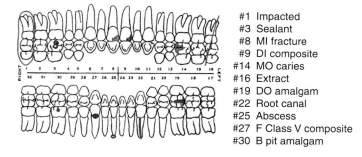

#1 Impacted
#3 Sealant
#8 MI fracture
#9 DI composite
#14 MO caries
#16 Extract
#19 DO amalgam
#22 Root canal
#25 Abscess
#27 F Class V composite
#30 B pit amalgam

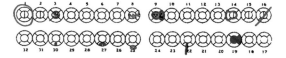

Charting

5

37

Examples of Charting Symbols II

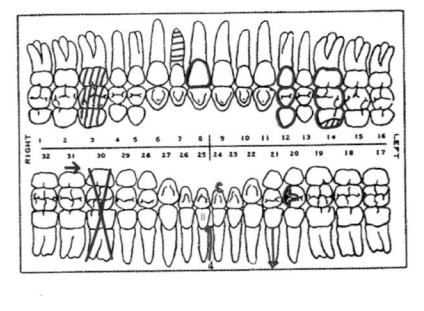

#3 Gold crown
#7 Implant
#8 Porcelain veneer
#12 Porcelain crown
#14 Porcelain fused to
metal crown
#20 MO porcelain inlay
#21 Root canal; apicoectomy
#24 Calculus on lingual
#25 4 mm MF perio pocket;
CLII mobility
#30 Missing
#31 Drifting mesially

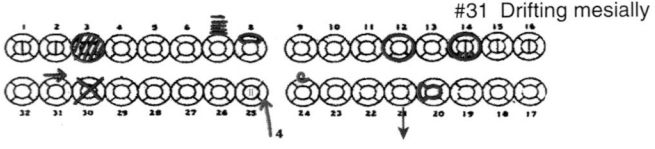

Common Charting Abbreviations

Adj	Adjustment	NC	No charge
Amal	Amalgam	NP	New patient
Anes	Anesthesia	OHI	Oral hygiene instruction
BA, NS	Broken appointment, no show	PA	Periapical
BWX	Bitewing x-ray	Pan, pano	Panoramic radiograph
Cr, crn	Crown	POT	Postoperative treatment (i.e., appointment following surgical procedure)
Dx	Diagnosis		
Epi	Epinephrine	Pro, prophy	Prophylaxis
Ext, TE	Extraction, tooth extraction	Pt	Patient
F/, /F	Full upper denture, full lower denture	RCT	Root canal therapy
FMX, FMS	Full mouth survey	RMH	Reviewed medical history
Imp	Impression	TX, Tx	Treatment
NA, NV	Next appointment, next visit		

Charting

5

Dental Terms and Abbreviations: Internet Resources

www.ada.org/sections/professionalResources/pdfs/dentalpractice_abbreviations.pdf
www.ada.org/glossaryforprofessionals.aspx

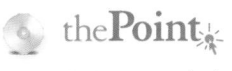 the**Point**

CD-ROM includes additional charting abbreviations, activities, and review for this chapter.

Clinical Dentistry Basics

Preparing and Positioning the Patient for Treatment Procedures

1. Before bringing the patient into the treatment room
   - review treatment plan and health history;
   - prepare instruments and materials for the procedure and place barriers;
   - place dental chair in upright position, raise chair arm, and clear patient's pathway of all equipment.
2. In the reception area, greet patient by name and introduce self.
3. Escort patient to treatment area and show the patient where to put personal items such as a purse or coat.
4. Seat patient and lower armrest.

5. Review health history with patient, take vital signs if required, put chart aside.

6. Provide brief explanation of the intended procedure, answer questions, and inform patient of approximate waiting time.

7. Place the patient's napkin; provide protective eyewear and mouthwash.

8. Wash hands, put on protective eyewear, mask and gloves.

9. Position patient for treatment and adjust the dental light to the treatment area.

10. Place handpiece(s), air/water syringe tips, and evacuation tips.

11. Position self: eye level 4" to 6" higher than dentist's, knees toward headrest of patient chair, thighs adjacent to patient's shoulder and parallel to the floor, and back straight (Figure 6-1).

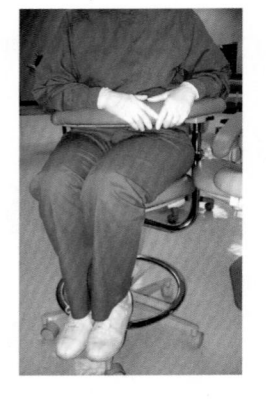

FIGURE 6–1 Dental assistant in position for chairside assisting.

Dismissing the Patient after Treatment Procedure

1. Slowly raise backrest to upright position and lift arm of chair.

2. Check patient's face for debris or smudges.

3. Remove the patient's napkin.

4. Move bracket table, light, and other objects out of pathway.
5. Remove gloves and mask, wash hands.
6. Provide posttreatment instructions.
7. Return personal items to client.
8. Assist patient in rising from chair, if needed.
9. Escort patient to reception desk and communicate patient's needs to business assistant.
10. Return to treatment room, put on mask and utility gloves to complete posttreatment aseptic procedures.

Instrument Transfer Basics

Instrument transfer occurs in the transfer zone, over the patient's chest in the 4 to 7 o'clock area. When working with a right-handed operator, the dental assistant transfers with the left hand. The dental assistant must anticipate each instrument needed and bring it to the dentist in the transfer zone. The dentist will signal for the next instrument by slightly moving the current instrument away from the treatment area without a change in his/her fulcrum or line of vision.

43

Clinical
Basics
6

One-Handed Instrument Transfer

After the patient is seated and the dentist is ready to begin the procedure

1. Simultaneously pass mirror and explorer, in position of use, to the operator. (Use a two-handed transfer for this—the mirror in your right hand and the explorer in your left.) Using your left hand, pick up the next instrument from dental tray.
2. Grasp instrument, on the handle away from the working end, between the thumb, index, and middle finger of the left hand.
3. Move instrument to transfer zone and direct the working end toward the arch being treated.
4. Remove explorer from dentist's hand with little finger of left hand (Figure 6-2). Instrument is removed distinctly and without hesitation.
5. Place pen grasp instrument in dentist's hand in position of use. Instrument is placed firmly and distinctly.
6. Instruments must be kept parallel to one another during transfer.
7. Return explorer to its original position on the dental tray. (If instruments are out of position on the tray, it is very difficult to quickly locate the needed instrument.) Or if that instrument will be needed again immediately, rotate instrument into passing position with one-handed technique.
8. Repeat process throughout procedure.

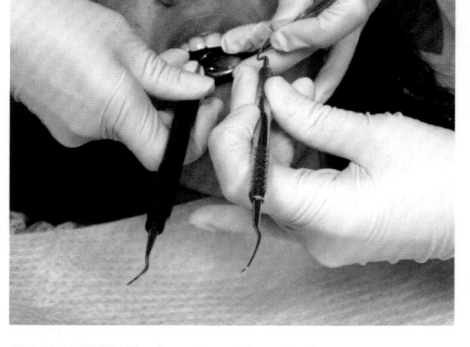

FIGURE 6–2 One-handed instrument transfer.

Moisture Control—Oral Evacuation Basics

1. Using a thumb-to-nose grasp, hold the high volume evacuation (HVE) in right hand when assisting a right-handed dentist (Figure 6-3). If dentist is left-handed, assistant will hold HVE in the left hand.

2. Place tip slightly posterior to the tooth under treatment.

3. Place tip opening parallel to the facial or lingual surface.

4. Rotate tip toward and beyond the incisal or occlusal surface.

   ■ For procedure on maxillary right posterior, place tip slightly distal, with opening parallel to lingual of tooth being treated.

   ■ For procedure on maxillary left posterior, place tip slightly distal, with opening parallel to buccal of tooth being treated.

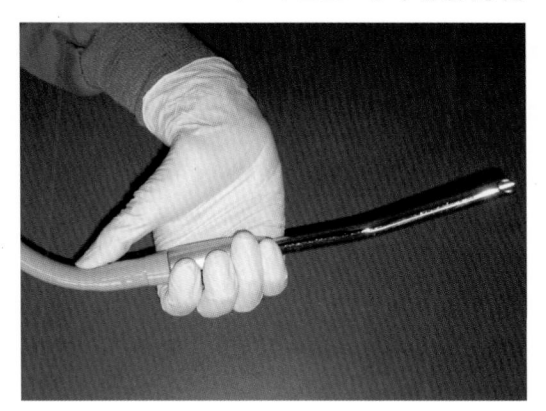

FIGURE 6-3 HVE thumb-to-nose grasp.

- For procedure on facial surface of maxillary or mandibular anterior area, place tip parallel to lingual of tooth being treated, with edge of tip slightly beyond incisal edge.

- For procedure on lingual surface of maxillary or mandibular anterior area, place tip parallel to facial of tooth being treated, with edge of tip slightly beyond incisal edge.

- For procedure on mandibular right posterior, place tip slightly distal, with opening parallel to lingual of tooth being treated.

- For procedure on mandibular left posterior, place tip slightly distal, with opening parallel to buccal of tooth being treated.

5. **DO NOT** place the tip on the soft palate, the center of the back of the tongue, or the soft tissue on the floor of the mouth.

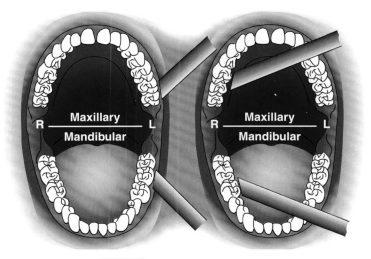

Clinical
Basics

6

Moisture Control and Isolation—Dental Dam Tray Setup

Purpose

To provide instrumentation for placing a barrier device for moisture control, patient protection, retraction, and reduction of microbes.

1. Dental dam template
2. Dental dam
3. Dental dam frame
4. Dental dam clamps
5. Floss
6. Applicator for lubricant
7. Dental dam punch
8. Dental dam clamp forceps
9. Iris scissors
10. Beavertail burnisher (Figure 6-5)

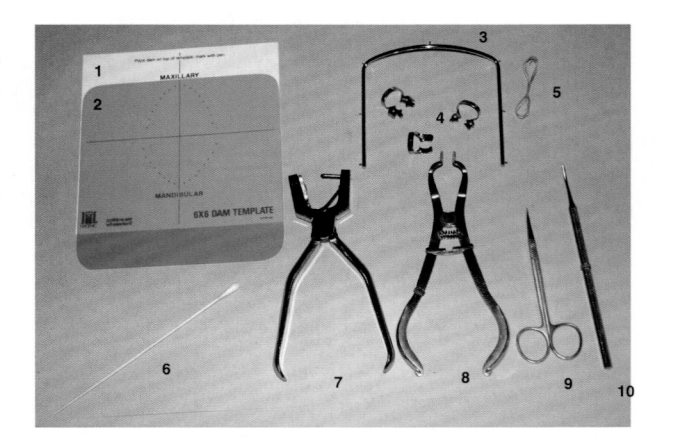

FIGURE 6–5 Dental dam tray setup.

Instruments and Materials Needed

Anesthetic syringe, anesthetic cartridge, and anesthetic needle.

Step-by-Step Procedure

1. Select the type of anesthetic. This is based on the treatment procedure to be performed and the patient's medical history as determined by the dentist.
2. Select the length (1" or 1⅝") and gauge (25, 27, or 30) of the needle. In general, longer and larger diameter (25 and 27) needles are used for mandibular block. Shorter and smaller diameter (30) needles are used for maxillary infiltration.
3. Insert the cartridge in the syringe: pull down on the thumb ring of the syringe, insert the rubber stopper end into the barrel of the syringe (Figure 6-6), and release the pressure on the thumb ring.

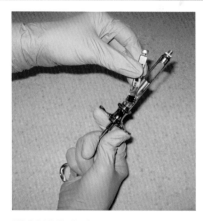

FIGURE 6–6 Loading the anesthetic cartridge.

Clinical
Basics

6

4. Place the needle on the syringe: remove the clear protective cap, push the exposed end of the needle through the opening in the hub of the anesthetic syringe (be careful to keep the needle straight so that it will pierce the rubber diaphragm in the aluminum cap of the cartridge), and screw the needle onto the hub.

5. Gently tap the bottom of the thumb ring to engage the harpoon in the rubber stopper of the cartridge.

6. Loosen and remove the colored needle cap.

7. Express a few drops of solution to ensure that the syringe is functioning properly.

8. Recap the needle using the one-handed scoop technique or a recapping device.

Replacing an Anesthetic Cartridge

1. Remove the empty cartridge: pull down on the thumb ring of the syringe, pull the cartridge down and away from the end of the needle, tilt the cartridge, and remove.

2. Insert the new cartridge in the syringe: pull down on the thumb ring of the syringe, insert the rubber stopper end into the barrel of the syringe, carefully align the center of the diaphragm with the end of the needle, and slide the cartridge into the end of the needle. Gently tap the bottom of the thumb ring to engage the harpoon in the rubber stopper.

Note: Never use a cartridge that is cracked or damaged. Never use one that has discolored or cloudy solution, an expired "use by" date, or an extruded rubber stopper.

Straight shank for straight, low-speed
handpiece

Latch shank for contra-angle
handpiece attachments

Friction grip shank for contra-angle
high-speed handpieces

Short shank friction grip also for
high-speed handpieces

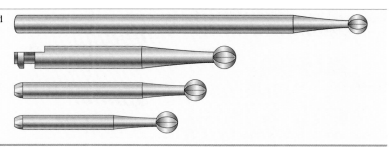

51

Clinical
Basics
6

Cavity Preparation Bur Shapes and Numbers

Round—1/2–8

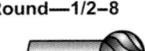

Inverted cone—33 1/2–37

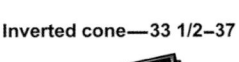

Pear—330

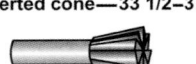

Straight fissure plain—56–58

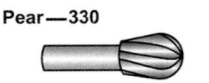

Straight fissure cross-cut—556–558

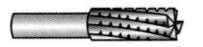

Tapered fissure plain—169–171

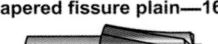

Tapered fissure cross-cut—699–702

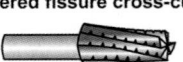

Round end fissure:

Straight plain 1156–1158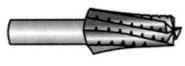

Straight cross-cut 1556–1558

Tapered plain 1169–1171

Tapered cross-cut 1700–1702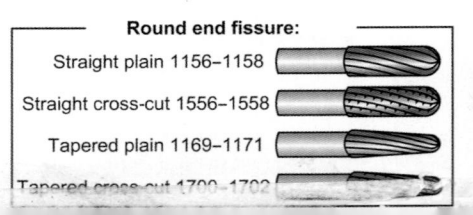

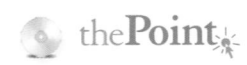

the**Point**

CD-ROM includes additional tray setups, activities, and review of the tray setups in this chapter.

Dental Radiography

Exposing Periapical Films with Bisecting Angle Technique

General Guidelines

- White side of film packet faces the lingual surface of the teeth.
- Dot toward the occlusal/incisal edge.
- Edge of film packet 1/8" beyond the occlusal/incisal edge.
- Anterior films placed vertically.

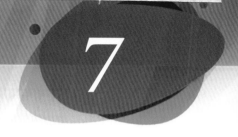

- Posterior films placed horizontally.
- Central ray is perpendicular to imaginary bisector.

If Using Preset Angulations

- Patient must be upright in the chair, midline perpendicular to the floor.
- For **maxillary and bitewing exposures**, the maxillary occlusal plane must be parallel to the floor.
- For **mandibular exposures**, mandibular occlusal plane must be parallel to the floor (Table 7-1).

TABLE 7-1 Recommended Angulations—Bisecting Angle Technique		
	Maxillary	**Mandibular**
Incisors	+40 to +45	–30
Canines	+45	–30 to –35
Premolars	+35	–15
Molars	+25	–10

Incisors

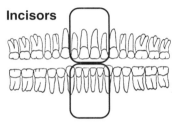

Canines

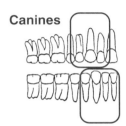

Premolars

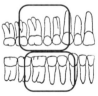

Molars

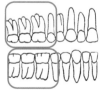

Exposing Horizontal Bitewings

General Guidelines

- Premolar bitewing—align the front edge of the film with the center of the mandibular canine.
- Molar bitewing—align the front edge of the film with the center of the mandibular 2nd premolar +10 vertical angulation.
- To avoid a cone-cut, align the position indicating device (PID) so that the bitewing tab is centered from top to bottom and from front to back.
- For correct horizontal angulation, place your finger along the facial surfaces of the posterior teeth and then place the PID so that the open end is parallel with your finger.

+10 vertical angulation

Premolars

Molars

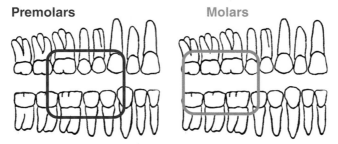

Dental
Radiography
7

Exposing Films with Paralleling Technique

General guidelines:

- White side of film packet faces the lingual surface of the teeth.
- Dot toward the slot of the film holder.
- Anterior films placed vertically.
- Posterior films placed horizontally.
- Place films away from the lingual toward center of oral cavity.
- Entire length of film must be parallel to the lingual surfaces of the teeth.

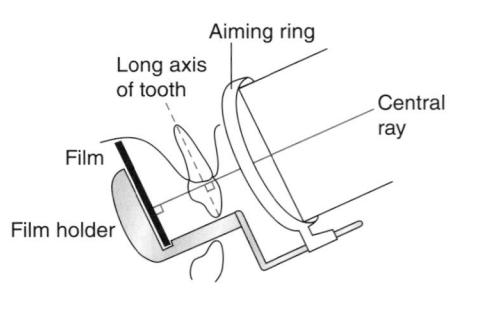

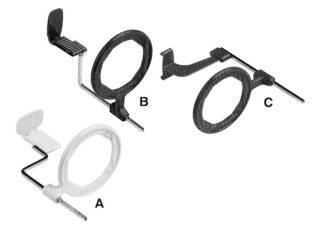

Rinn XCP (extension cone paralleling) instruments:
(A) posterior; (B) anterior; (C) bitewing.

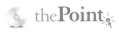 the Point

Assembling XCP film holders video on CD-ROM.

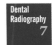

Dental
Radiography
7

Vertical Bitewings—Full Mouth Survey (Total of Seven Films)

Purpose

Examination of bone levels throughout the mouth with fewer films than full mouth periapical survey.

General Guidelines

- +10 vertical angulation.
- To avoid a cone-cut, align the PID so that the bitewing tab is centered from top to bottom and from front to back.
- For correct horizontal angulation, place your finger along the facial surfaces of the posterior teeth and then place the PID so that the open end is parallel with your finger.

Place Films and PID to Achieve the Following

1. Incisors: #1 film, vertical orientation—Central incisors centered on the film.
2. Canines: #1 film, vertical orientation—Canine is centered on the film. Interproximal spaces open on the mesial and distal of the canine.
3. Premolars: #2 film, vertical orientation—Distal portions of the canine crowns and all of the 1st premolar, 2nd premolar, and the mesial of the 1st molar crowns are visible. Interproximal spaces open, with emphasis on the maxillary canine/1st premolar and 1st premolar/2nd premolar areas.
4. Molars: #2 film, vertical orientation—All of the 1st molar, 2nd molar, and 3rd molar crowns or the crowns of the most distal tooth present are visible. Interproximal spaces open, with emphasis between maxillary 1st molar and 2nd molar.

Dental
Radiography
7

Vertical Bitewing Exposures—Film Placement

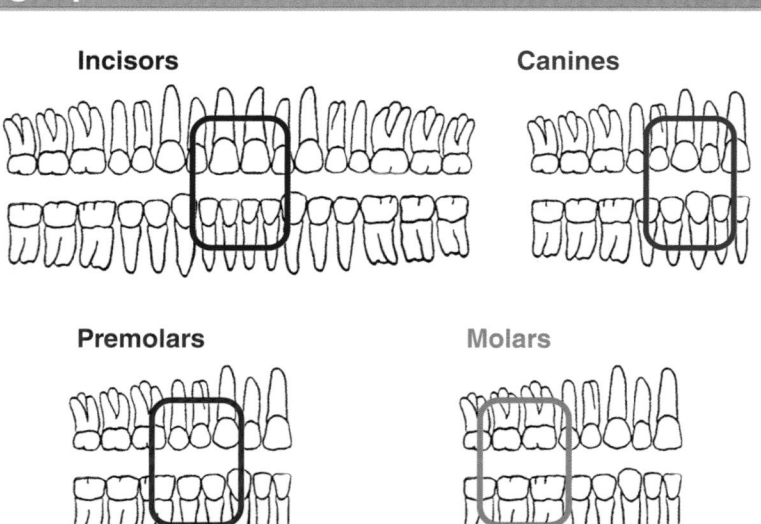

Incisors

Canines

Premolars

Molars

Radiographic Exposure

1. Put on dosimeter (film badge).
2. Wash hands.
3. Place barriers on exposure switch and work space.
4. Select the correct exposure settings required for the patient and exposure type.
5. Select appropriate positioning instruments.
6. Obtain the number of films required, cup for exposed films, and tissue for patient.
7. Seat patient and place the lead apron.
8. Wash hands and put on clean examination gloves.
9. Explain the procedure to the patient; communicate with the patient throughout procedure.
10. Place tubehead in close approximation to area for exposure before placing film.
11. Gently, but confidently, position film.
12. After each exposure, wipe saliva off the film packet and place them in the paper cup.

Dental
Radiography
7

63

After All Films Are Exposed

1. Remove gloves and wash hands.
2. Remove lead apron.
3. *Dismiss patient, put on utility gloves, remove barriers, clean and disinfect the treatment area.
4. *Wash and disinfect utility gloves, wash hands.

May be done at a later time if film exposure is part of another procedure.

Processing Films in Darkroom

1. Take films to darkroom.
2. Cover work surface with clean paper towel.
3. With gloved hands, open film packets and remove the inner paper packet; carefully open and drop the film out of this wrapping onto a dry surface without touching the film.
4. Place lead foil in container for proper disposal/recycling.
5. Discard contaminated film wraps into trash can.
6. Remove and discard gloves; **process films**.
7. Discard paper towel.

Processing Films in Automatic Processor with Daylight Loader

1. After removing treatment gloves, line the bottom of loader with a paper towel and place cup containing films and an empty cup into the daylight loader.
2. Put on clean examination gloves.
3. Insert hands into loader through ports.
4. Open film packets and remove the inner paper packet; carefully open and drop the film out of this wrapping onto a dry surface without touching the film.
5. Place empty packets and wrapping in the extra cup.
6. When all packets are opened, remove gloves and place in the paper cup.
7. Place film into processor slots, one film per slot.
8. After all films have been processed, withdraw hands from ports.
9. Reglove, open daylight loader, and remove trash, foil, and paper towel.
10. Discard waste appropriately.
11. Remove gloves and wash hands.

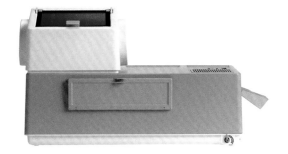

Air Techniques Peri-Pro III automatic processor with daylight loader.

Dental
Radiography
7

Steps in Manual Processing of Radiographs

1. Stir solutions and check temperature of developer. Adjust water temperature until developer is at 68°F.

2. At 68°F

   - Develop for 4½ minutes
   - Rinse for 30 seconds, slightly raise and lower rack in water continuously
   - Fix for 10 minutes
   - Wash for 20 minutes.

3. Replace unit cover between steps.

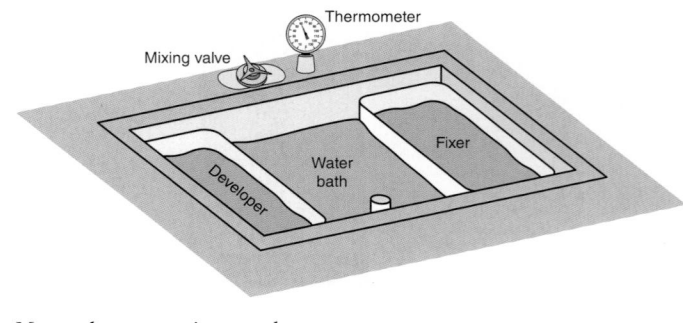

Manual processing tanks.

Mounting Dental Radiographs

1. Assemble equipment—film mount, processed radiographs, and viewbox.
2. Label the film mount with patient's name, dentist's name, and date.
3. Place all films on the work surface with the dot rounding up.
4. Locate the four bitewings (will have both maxillary and mandibular crowns on the film).
5. Mount the bitewings:
   - Bitewing closest to the center of the mount includes both premolars (Figure 7-1).
   - Bitewing closest to the outside of the mount includes all of the molars (Figure 7-2).
   - Occlusal plane curved as if smiling.
6. Locate the six anterior films (vertical films).

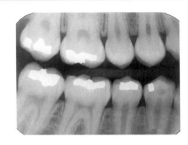

FIGURE 7–1 Premolar bitewing film.

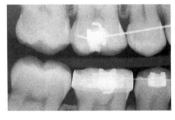

FIGURE 7–2 Molar bitewing film.

Dental
Radiography
7

7. Mount the anterior films:

- Maxillary incisors are larger than mandibular incisors (Figures 7-3 and 7-4).
- Maxillary cuspid is the longest tooth in the mouth.
- Place the incisal edge of the films toward the middle of the mount.

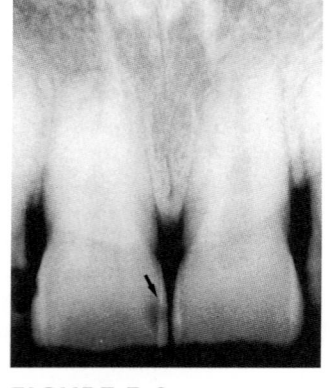

FIGURE 7–3 Maxillary incisor periapical film.

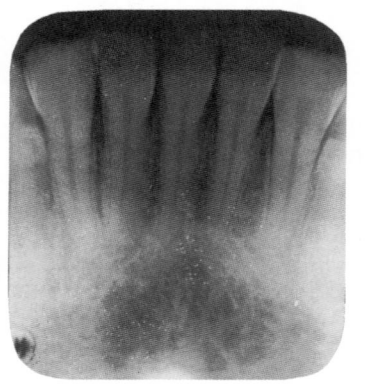

FIGURE 7–4 Mandibular incisor periapical film.

- Place the roots of the maxillary teeth toward the top and the roots of the mandibular teeth toward the bottom edges of the mount.

8. Locate the eight posterior films and mount.
   - Maxillary molars have three roots that are not clearly distinct (Figure 7-5).
   - Mandibular molars have two roots, a distinct mesial and a distal root (Figure 7-6).
   - Maxillary premolar and molar films will show the maxillary sinus.
   - Roots generally curve toward the distal.
   - Occlusal plane curved as if smiling.
   - Film closest to the center of the mount shows both premolars.
   - Film to the outside of the mount shows the 2nd and 3rd molar area.
   - Teeth on film oriented as in the mouth, the roots of maxillary teeth at the top and the roots of mandibular teeth at the bottom.

9. Review the entire mount for accuracy.

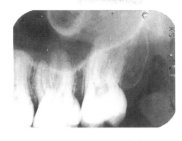

FIGURE 7–5 Maxillary molar periapical film.

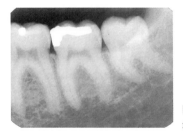

FIGURE 7–6 Mandibular molar periapical film.

Dental Radiography 7

Common Radiographic Errors

TABLE 7-2   Common Radiographic Errors

Error	Cause
Elongation	Too little vertical angulation
Foreshortening	Too much vertical angulation
Cone-cut	Partial exposure, PID opening not centered on film
Overlapping	Incorrect horizontal angulation
Distorted image	Bent film
Clear film	No x-rays reached the film
Dark/black film	Exposure to white light, overexposure, overdevelopment
Light film	Underexposure, underdevelopment
Herringbone pattern	Film placed with lead foil side next to lingual surface, reversed film
Fogged film	Exhausted chemicals, outdated film, light leaks

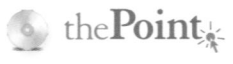
thePoint

CD-ROM includes activities and review for this chapter.

chapter

8

Dental Materials—Impression Materials

Alginate (Irreversible Hydrocolloid) Impression Material

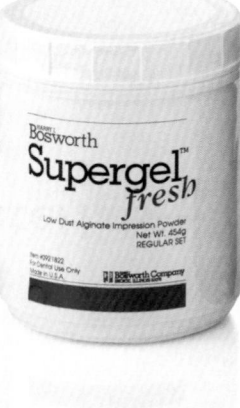
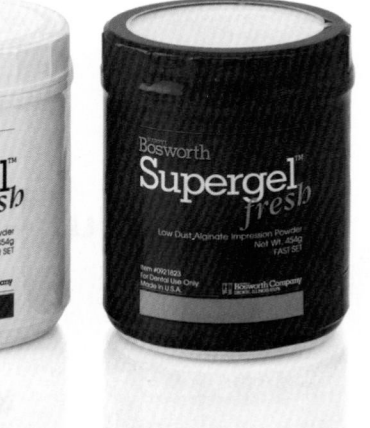

FIGURE 8–1 Supergel alginate. Image courtesy of Bosworth Company.

Uses

Fabrication of study models and working models for making appliances and custom impression trays.

Brand Names

Identic™, Integra™, Jeltrate®, Key-To®, Kromopan, Supergel®.

Clinical Considerations

- Alginate powder is supplied in canisters or bags.
- Use measuring scoop and water measure supplied by the manufacturer.
- In general, use two scoops for a mandibular impression and three scoops for a maxillary impression.
- Water temperature affects setting time.
- If taking impressions of both arches, prepare and take the mandibular impression first.
- Alginate is unstable, impressions will distort—pour in plaster/stone within 1 hour.

Impression
Materials
8

Step-by-Step Procedure—Taking an Alginate Impression

1. Assemble instruments and materials needed for procedure: impression trays, alginate spatula, mixing bowl, water measure, powder measure, alginate, patient cup, and mouthwash.
2. Seat patient in an upright position.
3. Wash hands and put on mask, protective eyewear, and gloves.
4. Explain the procedure to the patient.
5. Ask patient to rinse with mouthwash.
6. Try in tray(s) for proper fit. Tray must extend several millimeters beyond the central incisors to the retromolar area and facially into the vestibule to fit around the bone.
7. Measure water (room temperature) and pour into bowl.
8. Gently turn the canister over several times to fluff the alginate.
9. Measure alginate powder—scoop up powder, gently tap and level powder with alginate spatula.
10. Quickly incorporate all of the powder into the water using a circular motion, with the tip of the spatula toward the bottom of the bowl.
11. Spatulate for 30 to 45 seconds. Tilt the bowl toward you in the palm of your hand. Using a figure 8 motion, beat and press the alginate against the side of the bowl. Turn the bowl while you mix (Figure 8-2).
12. Gather the material together into a single mass.

13. Load the tray. For mandibular impressions, place one-half of the material on each side of the impression tray (Figure 8-3). Load the maxillary tray from the posterior with all of the alginate at once. Press down and spread over the entire surface of the tray.

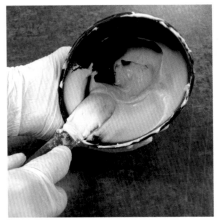

FIGURE 8–2 Mixing alginate.

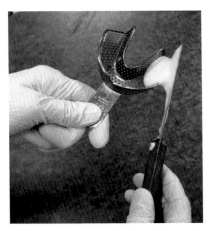

FIGURE 8–3 Loading alginate into impression tray.

Impression
Materials
8

14. Wet fingers and smooth material.
15. Dry the patient's teeth with A/W syringe or gauze.
16. Retract patient's right cheek.
17. Place the tray in the mouth. Leading with the posterior right corner of the tray, rotate the impression tray and center it over the teeth and arch.
18. Press tray firmly in place from posterior to anterior.
19. Gently pull the lips out and over the tray (mandibular—ask patient to raise tongue).

Note: To reduce gag reflex, have patient tilt their chin down, lean forward, and breathe through their nose.

20. Hold the tray in position until alginate is set (no longer tacky).
21. Grasp tray handle and remove impression with quick, firm pull.

Note: If it is difficult to remove the tray, a suction seal may have been created. Tilt tray handle to raise the posterior portion of the tray or place your finger under the periphery of the posterior portion of the tray on either side and lift gently.

22. Remove any debris from patient's face with moist cloth.

Postprocedure

1. Gently rinse the impressions under running water to remove any blood, saliva, or debris.
2. Spray with an approved surface disinfectant (iodophor or chlorine compound) and wrap in a moistened paper towel or place in a plastic bag.
3. After disinfection (10-minute contact with disinfectant), rinse with water and shake dry.
4. Unless pouring immediately, place in a sealed plastic bag labeled with the client's name.
5. Pour within 1 hour.

Uses

To obtain a dental impression for construction of casts for fabricating crowns, bridges, and partial and complete dentures (Figure 8-5).

Clinical Considerations

- Available in light (syringe), regular (syringe and/or tray), and heavy body (tray) viscosities.
- Supplied in two tubes, one base and one catalyst; some polyethers and polyvinyls are available in cartridges and mixing tips for use with a dispensing gun and also in magnums and mixing tips for use with an automixer (Figure 8-6).

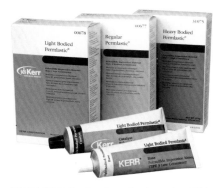

FIGURE 8–4 Permlastic polysulfide impression material in tubes. Image courtesy of Kerr Sybron.

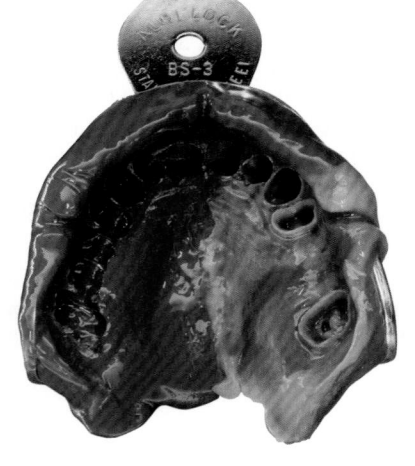

FIGURE 8–5 Elastomeric impression. Photo courtesy of 3M ESPE.

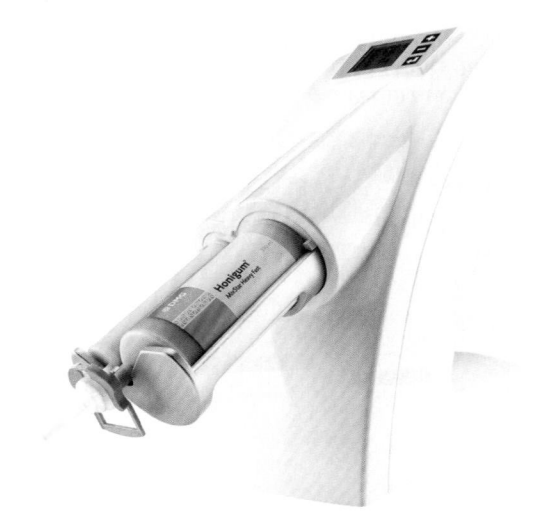

FIGURE 8–6 Automixer with impression material magnum and mixing tip. Image courtesy of DMG America.

- Requires a tray adhesive when using a custom tray.
- Setting time sensitive to temperature and moisture.

Preparation of Elastomeric Impression Materials Supplied in Tubes

1. Assemble instruments and materials: impression tray, impression syringe, impression material, tray adhesive, impression paste spatula, and heavy paper mixing pad (approx. 6" × 9") (Figure 8-7).
2. Extrude equal lengths of base and catalyst (close together, not touching) onto a paper pad.
3. With the tip of the spatula, use a spiral motion, working from top to bottom of the strips to mix the catalyst into the base very quickly (Figure 8-8).
4. Next use the flat side of the spatula to thoroughly mix the material in 30 to 45 seconds.
5. Load the syringe: using the back end of the syringe barrel, in short sweeping motions, scoop material up into the syringe until one-third full (Figure 8-9).

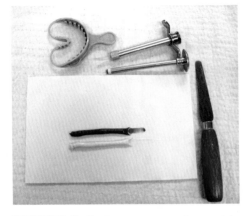

FIGURE 8–7 Instruments and materials for elastomeric impression.

Impression
Materials
8

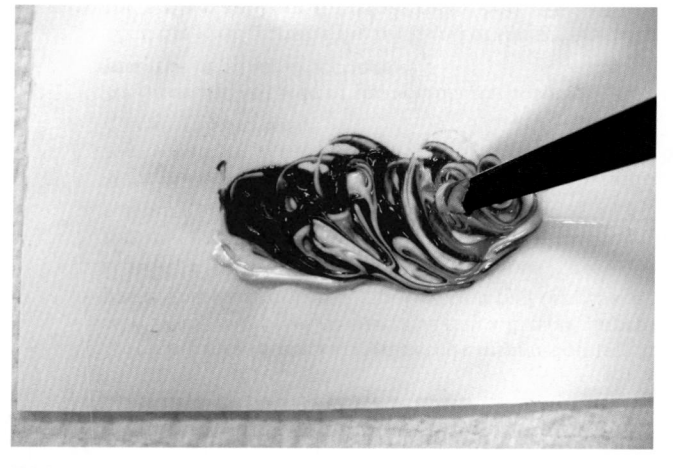

FIGURE 8–8 Incorporating base and catalyst.

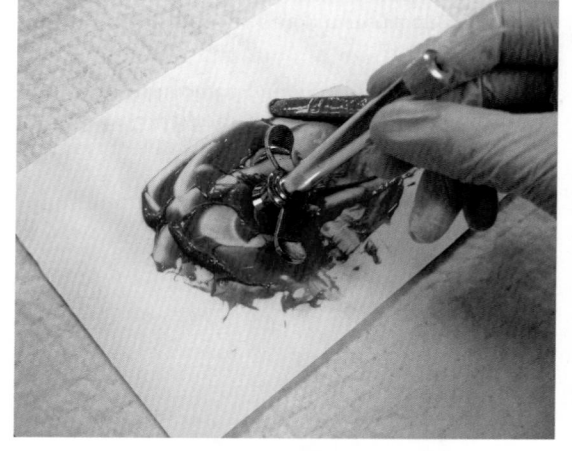

FIGURE 8–9 Loading the impression material syringe.

6. Place the plunger in the syringe barrel and extrude the material into the tip.

7. With blade of spatula, gather remainder of the impression material together and fill impression tray. Pass syringe and then impression tray to dentist.

8. The impression material will set in 6 to 10 minutes depending upon the type of material used.

Postprocedure

1. Disassemble the syringe

2. Remove excess material from the spatula and syringe. (When set, the material will be rubbery and will peel off the spatula and syringe. Brushes may be used to assist with cleaning the inside of the barrel of the syringe.) Clean and sterilize.

3. Tear off and dispose of top sheet of mixing pad.

4. Rinse impression with water, shake off excess moisture, and disinfect the impression (see Table 8-1).

5. After disinfection: rinse with water, shake to remove excess water, and place impression in a labeled, sealed bag for transport to the laboratory.

Impression
Materials
8

Disinfecting and Pouring Guidelines

TABLE 8-1   Disinfecting and Pouring Guidelines for Elastomeric Impression Materials

Elastomeric impression materials	Brand names (not an inclusive list)	Compatible disinfectants	Required contact time	Pour within
Polyether	Impregum, Polyjel NF	Spray with 1:213 iodophors or complex phenolics. Immerse in chlorine dioxide (3 min)	Spray and place in sealed bag for 10 min or immerse in chlorine dioxide for 3 min	1 wk
Polysulfide	COEFLEX, Permalastic	1:213 iodophors, glutaraldehydes, or complex phenolics	Spray and place in sealed bag or immerse for 10-30 min	2-3 h
Vinylpolysiloxane	Affinis, Aquasil, Cinch, Examix Extrude, Honigum, Imprint3, Virtual	1:213 iodophors, glutaraldehydes, or complex phenolics	Spray and place in sealed bag or immerse for 10-30 min	1 wk

Uses

To obtain impression of edentulous arches for construction of full dentures.

Brand Names

Coe-Flo™, Krex®, Opotow®, Superpaste™

Clinical Considerations

- Supplied in two tubes, one base and one catalyst.
- Setting time sensitive to temperature and moisture.
- Coating the patient's lip with petroleum jelly will prevent material from sticking and assist in cleanup.

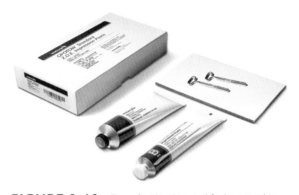

FIGURE 8–10 Permlastic zinc oxide impression material. Image courtesy of Waterpik Technologies.

Impression
Materials
8

Preparation of Zinc Oxide Eugenol Impression Material

1. Assemble instruments and materials: impression tray, impression material, tray adhesive, impression paste spatula, and heavy plastic-coated paper mixing pad (approx. 6" × 9").
2. Extrude equal lengths of base and catalyst (close together, not touching) onto a paper pad.
3. With the tip of the spatula, use a spiral motion, working from top to bottom of the strips to mix the catalyst into the base very quickly.
4. Next use the flat side of the spatula to thoroughly mix the material in 30 to 45 seconds.
5. With blade of spatula, gather impression material together and spread a thin, uniform layer in impression tray. Pass impression tray to dentist.
6. The impression material will set in 6 to 10 minutes depending upon the type of material used.
7. Remove excess cement from spatula before material sets up.

Postprocedure

1. Tear off and dispose of top sheet of mixing pad.
2. Rinse impression with water, shake off excess moisture, and disinfect the impression with iodophor (10-minute contact).
3. After disinfection: rinse with water, shake to remove excess water, and place impression in a labeled, sealed bag for transport to the laboratory.

Dental Materials—Cements

Dental Cements

Cements are classified both according to their use and according to their chemical properties. The dentist will choose a cement based on the characteristic required for a given procedure and situation.

Uses

1. Bases and liners—placed on the pulpal wall of the cavity preparation prior to restorative material to protect the pulp from thermal changes and to help the tooth recover from the trauma of decay and the irritation of the cavity preparation procedure.

2. Luting agents—adhere materials (i.e., crowns, bridges, orthodontic bands, and brackets) to tooth structures. There are different cements for both permanent and temporary luting (cementation).

3. Temporary restorations—soothing, short-term restorations that are relatively inexpensive and easy to place. Often used to restore tooth until the dentist is sure of the best treatment for the patient or to relieve discomfort until time is available to place a permanent restoration.

Types of Dental Cements

TABLE 9-1 Types of Dental Cements, Uses and Brand Names

Types of cements	Uses and brand names
Zinc oxide eugenol	Sedative base/liner—ZOE B&T, Cavitec
	Temporary restoration—IRM
	Temporary luting—Embonte, Temp-Bond
Calcium hydroxide	Cavity liner, especially with pulp exposures—Dycal, Life
Polycarboxylate	Permanent luting and insulating base—Durelon, LivCarbo, Tylok-Plus
Zinc phosphate	Permanent luting and insulating base—Fleck's zinc cement, Hy-Bond zinc
Glass ionomer	Base and liner—Fuji LINING, Vitrebond, KetacBond
	Permanent luting—Fuji CEM, Fuji I, Ketac-Cem, RelyX Luting
	Permanent restoration—Vitremer, Fuji IX, Riva, Ketac-Fil
Resin cement	Permanent luting—SpeedCEM, Calibra, SEcure, IntegraCem, Panavia F2.0
	Temporary luting—Neo-Temp

Dental
Cements
9

Mixing Zinc Oxide Eugenol (ZOE) Cement

1. Read manufacturer's instructions.

2. Fluff the powder in closed bottle, measure the powder with manufacturer's scoop, level with the cement spatula. Replace bottle cap immediately. (The amount of powder needed is determined by the amount of cement needed for the procedure.)

3. Draw up liquid into the dropper and replace the bottle cap immediately.

4. Holding the dropper perpendicular to the pad, dispense drops close to the powder without touching, one drop of liquid for each scoop of powder.

5. Divide the powder into two sections, next divide one section into two to three smaller sections.

6. Draw the larger section into liquid and incorporate the powder using a figure-of-8 motion, continue mixing in the smaller increments of powder until desired consistency is reached. Mixing time is 1 to 1½ minutes.

7. For temporary luting, the mix should be creamy and as the spatula is lifted off the pad, the cement should follow the spatula for about 1" before breaking into a thin thread.

8. For a base or temporary restoration, the cement should be puttylike and able to be rolled into a ball. (The dentist's preferences will also dictate the consistency required.)

9. Remove excess cement from the spatula with a 2 × 2 gauze.

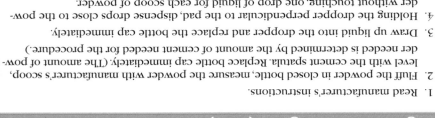

FIGURE 9–1 IRM zinc oxide eugenol cement. Image courtesy of Dentsply Caulk.

Mixing Polycarboxylate Cement

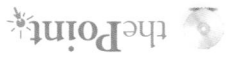

Mixing ZOE cement video on CD-ROM.

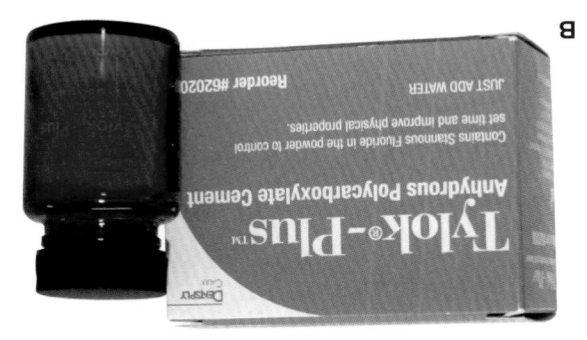

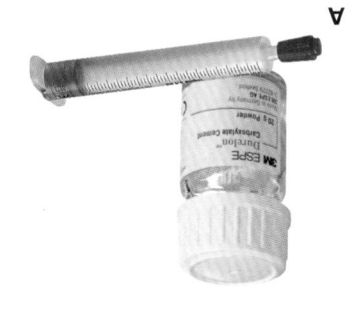

FIGURE 9-2 **(A)** Durelon carboxylate cement. **(B)** Tylok-Plus water-activated polycarboxylate cement. (A) Image courtesy of 3M ESPE. (B) Image courtesy of Dentsply Caulk.

1. Read the cement manufacturer's instructions.

2. Fluff the powder and measure powder with dispenser supplied by manufacturer.

3. Place the powder on the right side of the pad, replace cap on powder bottle.

4. Holding the liquid bottle or syringe perpendicular to the pad, dispense drops close to the powder without touching. Follow manufacturer's directions for the appropriate number of drops or calibrations per scoop of powder.

5. Incorporate all the powder into the liquid at once.

6. Mix quickly using a folding motion and some pressure (within 45 seconds).

7. For luting, the mix should be creamy and as the spatula is lifted off the pad, the cement should follow the spatula for about 1" before breaking into a thin thread. For a base, the liquid is decreased and the mix will be glossy, but the consistency is tacky and stiff.

8. Once mixing is completed, gather all material into one area, use immediately. Remove excess cement from the spatula with a moist 2 × 2 gauze.

9. For luting, use a plastic instrument to coat the internal surfaces of the crown or bridge. Transfer to the dentist occlusal side up.

10. For a base, hold the slab and a clean 2 × 2 gauze at the patient's chin and pass the plastic instrument to the dentist.

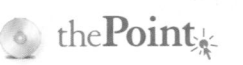 thePoint

Mixing polycarboxylate cement video on CD-ROM.

Mixing Glass Ionomer Cement

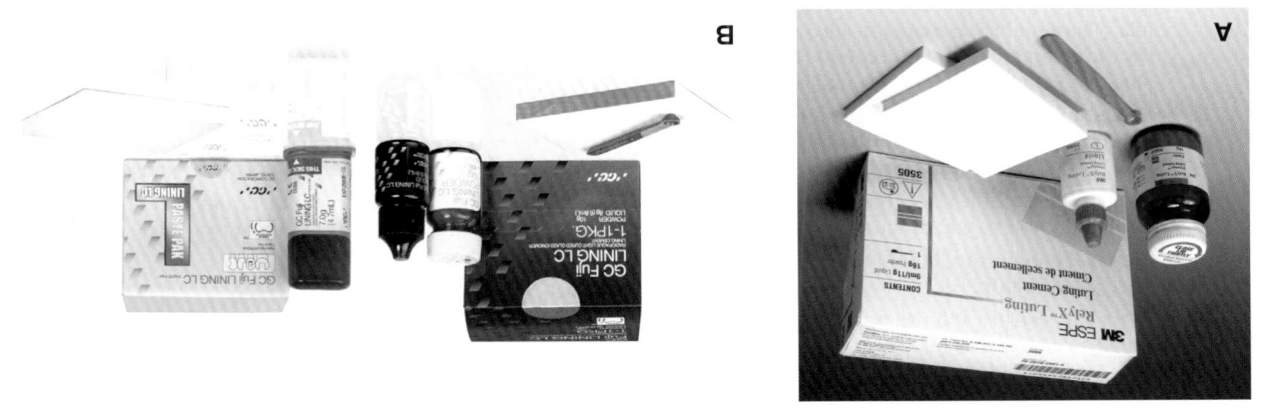

FIGURE 9-3 (A) RelyX glass ionomer permanent luting cement. (B) GC Fuji Lining glass ionomer cavity liner. (A) Image courtesy of 3M ESPE. (B) Image courtesy of GC America.

1. Read the manufacturer's instructions.
2. Fluff the powder in the closed bottle, measure the powder with scoop, and level with the cement spatula. (The amount of powder needed is determined by the amount of cement needed for the procedure and by the manufacturer's recommendations.)
3. Place the powder on the right side of the pad, replace cap on powder bottle.
4. Holding the dropper or liquid bottle perpendicular to the pad, dispense recommended amount of liquid close to the powder without touching.
5. Replace cap on the liquid immediately to prevent evaporation.
6. With the spatula, add the powder to the liquid in small, even increments.
7. Incorporate the powder using a figure-of-8 rotary motion and complete mixing in 60 seconds.
8. Once mixing is complete, gather all material into one area. Manipulation time is an additional 2 minutes while the surface of the cement remains glossy.
9. Remove excess cement from the spatula with a 2 × 2 gauze.
10. For luting, use a plastic instrument to thinly coat the internal surfaces of the crown or bridge. Transfer to the dentist occlusal side up.
11. If using glass ionomer as a base or restorative material, hold the slab and a clean 2 × 2 gauze at the patient's chin and pass the plastic instrument to the dentist.

Note: In addition to the powder/liquid form, glass ionomer cements are also available in two pastes and in premeasured capsules.

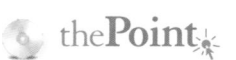 the**Point**

Mixing glass ionomer cement video on CD-ROM.

Mixing Zinc Phosphate Cement

1. Read the cement manufacturer's instructions.
2. Fluff the powder in the closed bottle.
3. Measure powder with dispenser supplied by the manufacturer.
4. Place powder on one end of a cooled glass slab, replace cap on powder bottle.
5. Holding the liquid bottle perpendicular to the pad, dispense drops at opposite end of slab. Follow manufacturer's directions for the appropriate number of drops per scoop of powder.
6. Divide the powder into four sections. Divide one of these into four smaller sections.
7. Add one small section into the liquid and mix in a sweeping figure-of-8 motion over a broad area for 15 seconds. Repeat for the remaining three small sections.
8. Next, mix in a larger ¼ section using the same motion and continue incorporating larger ¼ sections until the cement will string about 1" off the slab as the spatula is lifted (luting consistency).
9. For a base, mixing is the same but more powder is used until the material is very stringy.
10. Once mixing is completed, gather all material into one area, use immediately. Remove excess cement from the spatula with a moist 2 × 2 gauze.
11. For luting, use a plastic instrument to coat the internal surfaces of the crown or bridge. Transfer to the dentist occlusal side up.
12. For a base, roll cement into a ball using additional powder, pass to dentist on condenser tip.

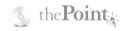 thePoint

Mixing zinc phosphate cement video on CD-ROM.

Dental
Cements

9

Resin Cement: Preparing the Cement, Abutment Tooth, and Restoration

1. Prepare internal surface of restoration for bonding with resin cement: metal restoration—micro-etch or sandblast; porcelain—etch or silanate

2. Remove provisional restoration, temporary cement, and debris from prepared tooth surfaces.

3. Rinse tooth and dry lightly with air or gauze.

4. Prime and bond the tooth surfaces according to the manufacturer's directions. (Self-adhesive resin cements eliminate the need for pretreating the tooth with prime and bond agents.)

5. To facilitate cleanup, apply a separating medium (KY jelly, petroleum jelly, and glycerine) to exterior surfaces of restoration, adjacent teeth, and gingiva.

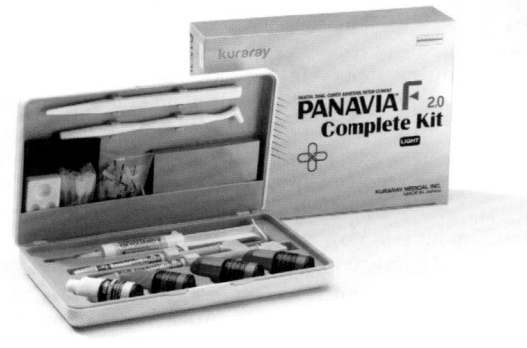

FIGURE 9–4 Panavia F2.0 resin permanent luting cement. Image courtesy of Kuraray America Co.

6. Dispense equal amounts of base paste and catalyst paste onto mixing pad, mix for 20 to 30 seconds; remove excess cement from spatula; use a plastic instrument to coat the internal surfaces of the restoration; pass restoration to dentist for seating.

7. Remove gross excess cement at gingival margin with super floss, explorer, or scaler.

8. Wait for a complete self-cure or light cure before final removal of cement and occlusal adjustment.

Cement Cleanup and Disinfection

Remove cement from mixing and placement instruments with an alcohol-moistened gauze as soon as possible. Hardened cement is very difficult to remove. A baking soda solution or using the ultrasonic with a commercial cement removal solution may help.

Cement bottles, dispensing scoops, and syringes must be properly disinfected after use. Mixing and placement instruments should be sterilized. Glass or plastic slabs that can be sterilized are preferred. Paper mixing pads are convenient but are a source of contamination.

Varnishes, Dentin Sealants, and Desensitizers

Varnishes, dentin sealants, and desensitizers are non-cement, liquid agents used to seal the dentin, reduce sensitivity, and protect the pulp from chemical irritation. These do not require mixing and are applied to cavity walls or exposed dentin with a disposable plastic brush or with a small cotton pellet (Figure 9-5).

Brand Names

Barrier, Copaliner Varnish, Gluma, HemaSeal & Cide, Seal & Protect, Systemp, Zarosen.

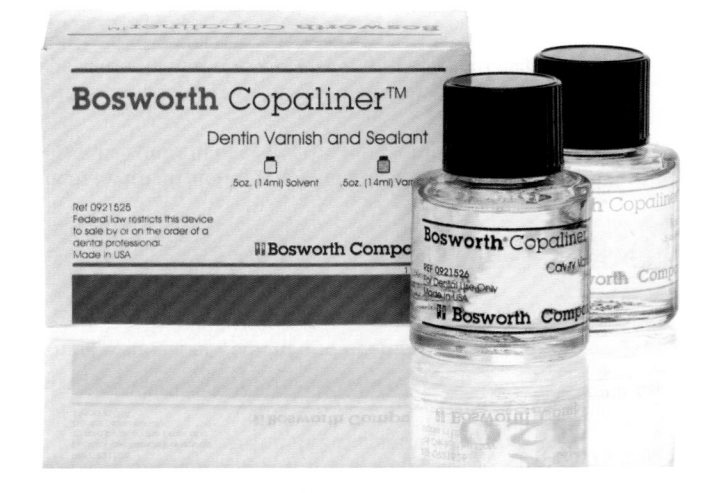

FIGURE 9–5 Dentin sealant. Image courtesy of Bosworth Company.

Dental Materials—Product Names, Material Types, and Manufacturers

Table 10-1 lists many common dental materials alphabetically by brand name. The table includes a description of the type of material and specifies the manufacturer.

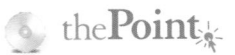

On the companion CD-ROM, you can search for dental materials by type of material, manufacturer, or brand name. The CD also includes images for most of these materials and provides a link to the manufacturer's web site.

TABLE 10-1

Brand name	Type of dental material	Manufacturer
AdheSE®	Bonding adhesive, self-etch	Ivoclar Vivadent Inc.
Adper™ Prompt L-Pop™	Bonding adhesive system, one-step self-etch unit dose	3M ESPE
Adper™ Scotch Bond™	Bonding adhesive, multiple component self-etch	3M ESPE
Affinis®	Impression material, vinyl polysiloxane (VPS)	Coltene Whaledent
Algin•X™ Ultra	Alginate alternative impression material	DENTSPLY Caulk
AlgiNot	Alginate alternative impression material	Kerr Sybron Dental Specialties
AMALGAMBOND® Plus	Bonding adhesive for amalgam and composite	Parkell, Inc.

Brand name	Type of dental material	Manufacturer
Amelogen Plus	Composite restorative, light cure	Ultradent Products, Inc.
Apexit® Plus	Endodontic sealer paste	Ivoclar Vivadent Inc.
Aquasil Ultra	Impression material, VPS	DENTSPLY Caulk
Barricaid®	Periodontal dressing, light cure	DENTSPLY Caulk
Barrier	Cavity varnish/dentin sealant	Waterpik Technologies
Biocide G30™	High-level disinfectant/sterilant immersion solution	Biotrol
Birex	Surface disinfectant—phenol	Biotrol
Blu-Mousse®	Impression material/bite registration paste	Parkell, Inc.
Calibra®	Permanent luting cement, resin	DENTSPLY Caulk
Carbocaine	Local anesthetic	Carestream Health, Inc.
CaviCide®	Surface disinfectant—synergized quaternary	Kerr TotalCare
Cavit™	Temporary filling material, no mix	3M ESPE
Cavitec™	Cavity liner/base, zinc oxide eugenol (ZOE)	Kerr Sybron Dental Specialties
CavityShield™	Fluoride varnish	3M ESPE

(Continued)

Dental
Materials
10

TABLE 10-1 *(Continued)*

Brand name	Type of dental material	Manufacturer
Ceram X™	Composite restorative, nano-ceramic light cure	DENTSPLY Caulk
Cinch™	Impression material, VPS	Parkell, Inc.
Citanest®	Local anesthetic	DENTSPLY Pharmaceuticals
ClearFil™ SE Protect	Bonding adhesive, self-etch light cure	Kuraray America Co.
Clinpro™ Sealant	Pit and fissure sealant, fluoride releasing	3M ESPE
COECIDE™ XL	High-level disinfectant/sterilant immersion solution	GC America
COEFLEX®	Impression material, polysulfide	GC America
COE-FLO™	Impression material, ZOE	GC America
COE-PAK™	Periodontal dressing	GC America
Compoglass®	Compomer restorative (glass ionomer and composite)	Ivoclar Vivadent Inc.
Conseal F	Pit and fissure sealant, fluoride releasing	Southern Dental Industries
Consepsis	Antimicrobial solution for prepared tooth surfaces	Ultradent Products, Inc.
Contour™	Amalgam restorative	Kerr Sybron Dental Specialties
Copaliner®	Cavity varnish/dentin sealant	Bosworth Company

Brand name	Type of dental material	Manufacturer
Copalite® Varnish	Cavity varnish/dentin sealant	Cooley & Cooley, Ltd.
Dimension™	Impression material, VPS	3M ESPE
Dispersalloy®	Amalgam restorative	DENTSPLY Caulk
DuoTemp™	Temporary filling material, eugenol free, dual cure	Coltene Whaledent
Durelon™	Permanent luting cement, polycarboxylate	3M ESPE
Dycal®	Cavity liner/base, calcium hydroxide	DENTSPLY Caulk
Dyract®	Compomer restorative (glass ionomer and composite)	DENTSPLY Caulk
Esthet•X®	Composite restorative, light cure	DENTSPLY Caulk
EXABITE™ II	Bite registration paste	GC America
EXAMIX™	Impression material, VPS	GC America
ExciTE® F	Bonding adhesive, light cure single component	Ivoclar Vivadent Inc.
Expasyl®	Gingival retraction paste material	Kerr Sybron Dental Specialties
Extrude®	Impression material, VPS	Kerr Sybron Dental Specialties
Fermit®	Temporary filling material, light cure	Ivoclar Vivadent Inc.

(Continued)

TABLE 10-1 (Continued)

Brand name	Type of dental material	Manufacturer
Filtek™	Composite restorative, light cure	3M ESPE
Fleck's Zinc	Permanent luting cement, zinc phosphate	Keystone Industries
Flexitime®	Impression material, VPS	Heraeus Kulzer
Fynal®	Permanent luting cement, ZOE	DENTSPLY Caulk
G-aenial™ Bond	Bonding adhesive, one-step self-etch	GC America
GC Fuji I®	Permanent luting cement, glass ionomer	GC America
GC Fuji II™	Glass ionomer restorative	GC America
GC Fuji IX™ GP	Glass ionomer restorative, packable posterior	GC America
GC Fuji LINING™	Cavity liner/base, glass ionomer	GC America
GC Fuji TRIAGE®	Pit and fissure sealant, fluoride releasing	GC America
GC TEMP ADVANTAGE®	Temporary luting cement, non-ZOE	GC America
G-CEM™	Permanent luting cement, self-adhesive resin	GC America
Geristore®	Compomer restorative (glass ionomer and composite)	DenMat Holdings, LLC
Getz® Blue Core	Crown buildup material	Waterpik Technologies

Brand name	Type of dental material	Manufacturer
Glacier	Composite restorative, light cure	Southern Dental Industries
Gluma®	Desensitizing dentinal sealer	Heraeus Kulzer
go!	Bonding adhesive, single-component self-etch	Southern Dental Industries
GRADIA® DIRECT	Composite restorative, microfilled hybrid light cure	GC America
Heliomolar®	Composite restorative, light cure	Ivoclar Vivadent Inc.
Helioseal F	Pit and fissure sealant, fluoride releasing	Ivoclar Vivadent Inc.
Hemaseal & Cide	Antimicrobial desensitizer—used after etch before bond	Advantage Dental Products, Inc.
Hemodent™	Hemostatic liquid	Premier
Herculite™ Ultra	Composite restorative, light cure	Kerr Sybron Dental Specialties
Honigum	Impression material, VPS	DMG America
Hydrosil®	Impression material, VPS	DENTSPLY Caulk
Hydrox®	Cavity liner/base, calcium hydroxide	Bosworth Company
iBond®	Bonding adhesive, single component	Heraeus Kulzer

(Continued)

TABLE 10–1 *(Continued)*

Brand name	Type of dental material	Manufacturer
Impregum™	Impression material, polyether	3M ESPE
Imprint™ 3	Impression material, VPS	3M ESPE
Infinity®	Permanent luting cement, resin ionomer	DenMat Holdings, LLC
IntegraBond™	Bonding adhesive, single component	Premier
IntegraCem™	Permanent luting cement, resin dual cure	Premier
Integrity™	Provisional cr & br material	DENTSPLY Caulk
IRM®	Temporary filling material, ZOE	DENTSPLY Caulk
Jeltrate®	Alginate impression material	DENTSPLY Caulk
Kalginate®	Alginate impression material	Waterpik Technologies
KALORE™	Composite restorative, nano-hybrid light cure	GC America
Ketac™ Bond	Cavity liner/base cement, glass ionomer	3M ESPE
Ketac™ Cem	Permanent luting cement, glass ionomer	3M ESPE
Ketac™ Fil/Molar	Glass ionomer restorative	3M ESPE
Ketac™ Nano	Glass ionomer restorative, resin modified	3M ESPE

Brand name	Type of dental material	Manufacturer
Ketac™ Silver	Glass ionomer restorative, silver reinforced	3M ESPE
Key-To®	Alginate impression material	Waterpik Technologies
Kolorz ClearShield	Fluoride varnish	DMG America
Kool-Dam™	Gingival barrier material, light cure	Pulpdent
Krex®	Impression material, ZOE	Waterpik Technologies
Life™	Cavity liner/base, calcium hydroxide	Kerr Sybron Dental Specialties
Lime-Lite™	Cavity liner, light cure calcium hydroxide	Pulpdent
Luxatemp	Provisional cr & br material	DMG America
Marcaine	Local anesthetic	Carestream Health, Inc.
Maxcem Elite™	Permanent luting cement, self-adhesive resin	Kerr Sybron Dental Specialties
MetaSEAL™	Endodontic sealer, dual cure	Parkell, Inc.
Miracle Mix®	Glass ionomer restorative, metal reinforced	GC America
Multilink® Automix	Permanent luting cement, self-curing resin	Ivoclar Vivadent Inc.
Neo-Temp®	Temporary luting cement, resin	Waterpik Technologies
One Coat 7.0	Bonding adhesive, single-component self-etch	Coltene Whaledent

(Continued)

Dental
Materials
10

TABLE 10-1 *(Continued)*

Brand name	Type of dental material	Manufacturer
Opotow®	Impression material, ZOE	Waterpik Technologies
Opotow® Trial Cement	Temporary luting cement, ZOE	Waterpik Technologies
OptiBond™ All-In-One	Bonding adhesive, self-etch single component	Kerr Sybron Dental Specialties
OptiBond™ Solo Plus	Bonding adhesive, light cure single component	Kerr Sybron Dental Specialties
Opti-Cide³®	Surface disinfectant—isopropanol	Biotrol
OptiGuard®	Composite surface sealant	Kerr Sybron Dental Specialties
Panavia F2.0	Permanent luting cement, self-adhesive resin	Kuraray America Co.
Peridex™	Antimicrobial oral rinse (chlorhexidine gluconate)	3M ESPE
PerioCare®	Periodontal dressing	Pulpdent
Permite	Amalgam restorative	Southern Dental Industries
Permlastic®	Impression material, polysulfide	Kerr Sybron Dental Specialties
PIP	Pressure indicating paste to locate pressure areas on interior of denture	Keystone Industries
Plastopaste™	Impression material, ZOE	Bosworth Company

Brand name	Type of dental material	Manufacturer
Polyjel® NF™	Impression material, polyether	DENTSPLY Caulk
Prime & Bond® NT™	Bonding adhesive, single component	DENTSPLY Caulk
ProCide-D Plus	High-level disinfectant/sterilant immersion solution	Kerr TotalCare
Prodigy™	Composite restorative, light cure	Kerr Sybron Dental Specialties
Protemp™ Plus	Provisional cr & br material	3M ESPE
Racellets®	Hemostatic pellets to control bleeding at gingival margin	Pascal
RC Prep®	Endodontic intracanal chelating agent/lubricant	Premier
Regisil®	Bite registration paste	DENTSPLY Caulk
RelyX™	Permanent luting cement, glass ionomer	3M ESPE
RelyX™ Unicem	Permanent luting cement, self-adhesive resin	3M ESPE
Reprosil™	Impression material, VPS	DENTSPLY Caulk
Scotchbond™	Bonding adhesive, multiple component	3M ESPE
SEcure™	Permanent luting cement, resin	Parkell, Inc.
Seek	Caries indicator solution	Ultradent Products, Inc.

(Continued)

Dental
Materials
10

TABLE 10-1 *(Continued)*

Brand name	Type of dental material	Manufacturer
SeT	Permanent luting cement, self-adhesive resin	Southern Dental Industries
SmartCem™2	Permanent luting cement, self-adhesive resin	DENTSPLY Caulk
SmarTemp®	Provisional cr & br material	Parkell, Inc.
Snoop™	Caries detecting dye	Pulpdent
SpeedCEM®	Permanent luting cement, resin self-adhesive	Ivoclar Vivadent Inc.
Status Blue	Alginate alternative impression material	DMG America
Styptin	Hemostatic solution—aluminum chloride	DUX Dental
Superbite™	Bite registration paste, ZOE	Bosworth Company
Supergel®	Alginate impression material	Bosworth Company
Synergy® D6	Composite restorative, light cure	Coltene Whaledent
TempBond®	Temporary luting cement, ZOE	Kerr Sybron Dental Specialties
Tenure® Uni-Bond	Bonding adhesive, self-etch	DenMat Holdings, LLC
Tetric®	Composite restorative, light cure	Ivoclar Vivadent Inc.
TPH®3	Composite restorative, light cure	DENTSPLY Caulk

Brand name	Type of dental material	Manufacturer
Traxodent®	Hemostatic retraction paste	Premier
Tylok® Plus	Permanent luting cement, polycarboxylate	DENTSPLY Caulk
Tytin™	Amalgam restorative	Kerr Sybron Dental Specialties
Ultra-Bond® Plus	Permanent luting cement, resin	DenMat Holdings, LLC
UltraSeal XT Plus	Pit and fissure sealant, fluoride releasing	Ultradent Products, Inc.
Valiant®	Amalgam restorative	Ivoclar Vivadent Inc.
Vanish™	Fluoride varnish	3M ESPE
Venus®	Composite restorative, light cure	Heraeus Kulzer
Vertise™ Flow	Composite restorative, self-adhering light cure	Kerr Sybron Dental Specialties
Virtual®	Impression material, VPS	Ivoclar Vivadent Inc.
Virtuoso®	Composite restorative, light cure	DenMat Holdings, LLC
ViscoStat	Hemostatic solution	Ultradent Products, Inc.
Vitrebond™	Cavity liner/base, glass ionomer	3M ESPE
Vitremer™	Glass ionomer core buildup/restorative cement	3M ESPE

(Continued)

Dental
Materials
10

TABLE 10–1 *(Continued)*

Brand name	Type of dental material	Manufacturer
Wave	Composite restorative, flowable light cure	Southern Dental Industries
Xeno® IV	Bonding adhesive, self-etch	DENTSPLY Caulk
XP Bond™	Bonding adhesive, total etch	DENTSPLY Caulk
Xylocaine®	Local anesthetic	DENTSPLY Pharmaceuticals
Z100™	Composite restorative, light cure	3M ESPE
Zarosen	Desensitizing dentinal sealer	Cetylite Industries, Inc.
ZONE	Temporary luting cement, non-ZOE	DUX Dental

Laboratory Materials and Procedures

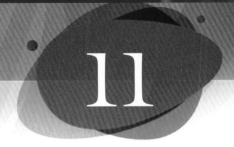

Fabricating a Dental Model

Assemble Equipment and Materials Needed for Procedure

Flexible mixing bowl, plaster spatula, graduated water cylinder, dental plaster or stone, scale, vibrator, plastic barrier, paper towels, impression, and plastic or glass slab/tile

Water/Powder Ratio

30 mL water/100 g stone (for art base 45 mL water/150 g stone)

50 mL water/100 g plaster (for art base 75 mL water/150 g plaster)

Step-by-Step Procedure—Pouring the Impression with Plaster/Stone

1. Place plastic cover over top of vibrator.
2. Wash hands and put on mask, protective eyewear, and gloves.
3. Gently dry impression with A/W syringe.
4. Measure water and pour it into a flexible mixing bowl.
5. Place towel on scale and weigh out stone or plaster.
6. Pick up the towel and gradually slide the stone/plaster into the water.
7. Stir the water and powder together and mix for 30 to 60 seconds by pressing the spatula against the side of the bowl. Do not whip (whipping incorporates air bubbles).
8. Turn the vibrator to low or medium speed.
9. Place the mixing bowl on the vibrator; press down and rotate the bowl to bring bubbles to the surface. (Mixing and vibrating should be completed in less than 2 minutes.)
10. Pick up the impression and place the edge of the tray (edge close to the handle) on the vibrator.

11. With the spatula, place a small amount of plaster/stone in the posterior area on one side of the dental arch (Figure 11-1).

12. Tilt the tray to allow the plaster/stone to flow into the teeth around the arch.

13. Continue adding small increments until all tooth areas of the impression are covered.

14. Add larger increments until the entire impression is filled.

15. Place the remaining plaster/stone on a glass slab or tile and shape into a base approximately the same size as the impression tray and ½" to 1" thick (Figure 11-2).

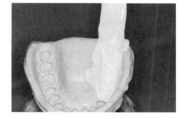

FIGURE 11–1 Pouring a dental model. Reprinted with permission from Gladwin MA, Bagby M. *Clinical Aspects of Dental Materials: Theory, Practice, and Cases*. 3rd ed. Baltimore, MD: Lippincott Williams & Wilkins; 2008.

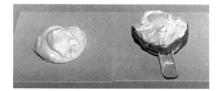

FIGURE 11–2 Plaster base and poured impression. Reprinted with permission from Gladwin MA, Bagby M. *Clinical Aspects of Dental Materials: Theory, Practice, and Cases*. 3rd ed. Baltimore, MD: Lippincott Williams & Wilkins; 2008.

Lab
Procedures
11

16. Invert the filled impression onto the base without pushing into the base.

17. Hold the impression by the handle to keep it level while smoothing the base mix up into the inverted material. Do not cover the edges of the impression tray or the tray will be locked in when the plaster hardens.

18. Place any excess plaster in a trash container.

19. Clean and disinfect plaster bowl and spatula.

20. Allow the model to set for 1 hour before separating.

21. To separate, use a lab knife to remove any excess plaster from around the margins of the impression tray.

22. Raise the anterior portion of the tray to loosen slightly and then pull straight up on the tray handle to remove impression from the model.

Fabricating a Vacuum-Formed Bleaching Tray or Night Guard

Equipment and Instruments Needed

Thermoplastic sheet (0.035/0.040 for bleaching and 0.080/0.150 for night guards or mouth guards), block-out material, curing light, small curved scissors, micro torch, and vacuum forming unit.

Preprocedure

1. Pour impression on stone. Place stone in tooth-bearing areas only. Model should be U-shaped.
2. After model is set, remove from impression and trim model as close as possible without cutting teeth.

Step-by-Step Procedure

1. For bleaching trays, place block-out resin on the facial surfaces of the teeth (not more than 1 mm

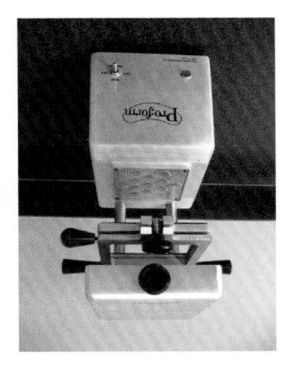

FIGURE 11-3
Thermoplastic sheets and trimmed model with block-out resin.

thick) to create a space to hold the bleaching material. Do not cover the occlusal or incisal surfaces, and keep the block-out resin 1 mm away from the gingiva. Light cure the block-out resin.

2. Place acrylic sheet of the appropriate thickness in the frame of the unit, screw it shut, and raise it to start position (Figure 11-4).

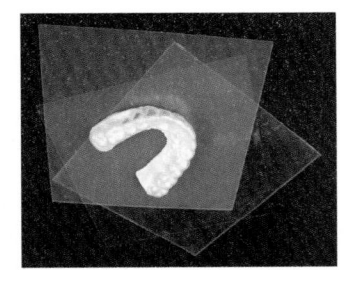

FIGURE 11-4
Vacuum forming unit.

3. Place heating element directly above the frame.
4. Center the prepared model on the vacuum forming unit platform.
5. Heat the resin material until it sags approximately 1" below the frame.
6. Turn on the vacuum and pull the frame down over the model. Keep vacuum on for 1 minute.
7. Turn off the vacuum and heater. Swing the heating element to the side.
8. Allow the resin to cool before removing from the frame.
9. Trim the excess resin from around the model and separate.
10. Trim the tray to the desired form (For bleaching trays, the tray border should be 0.5 mm from the gingival margin.) (Figure 11-5).
11. Replace the tray on the model. Lightly flame the edges of the tray with the micro torch and smooth with moist fingers.

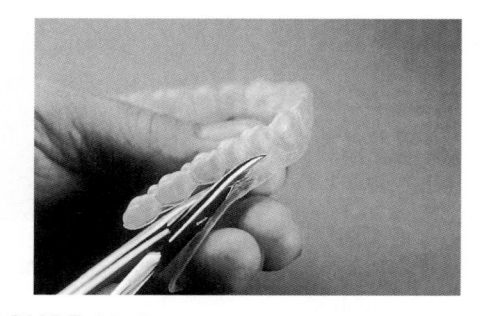

FIGURE 11–5 Trimming a bleaching tray. Reprinted with permission from Gladwin MA, Bagby M. *Clinical Aspects of Dental Materials: Theory, Practice, and Cases*. 3rd ed. Baltimore, MD: Lippincott Williams & Wilkins; 2008.

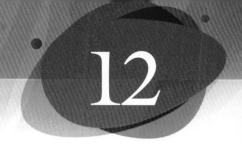

chapter

12

Clinical Procedures

This chapter outlines the basic steps in many of the procedures performed in general dentistry practices. The procedural steps are listed in the column on the left and the instruments and materials necessary for each step are listed in the column on the right.

The tray setups for these procedures are pictured in Chapter 13.

Clinical procedures included in this chapter:

1. Cavity Preparation and Amalgam Restoration
2. Cavity Preparation and Composite Restoration
3. Crown and Bridge Preparation
4. Crown and Bridge Cementation/Bonding
5. Root Canal
6. Basic Extraction
7. Multiple Extractions and Alveoplasty/Gingivoplasty
8. Impacted Tooth Extraction

Cavity Preparation and Amalgam Restoration

Step-by-step procedure	Instruments and materials used
1. Examine oral cavity	1. Basic setup
2. Administer topical and local anesthesia	2. Anesthesia setup
3. Place dental dam (optional)	3. Dental dam setup
4. Remove decay and prepare cavity	4. Handpiece (HP) burs, spoon, hand-cutting instrument
5. Place matrix (if Class 2 cavity)	5. Matrix band, retainer, wedge
6. Apply base and/or dentin sealant/varnish	6. Applicator, mixing pad
7. Place amalgam	7. Carrier and condenser
8. Carve amalgam	8. Hollenback, discoid–cleoid, burnisher
9. Remove matrix	9. Hemostat, cotton pliers

Step-by-step procedure	Instruments and materials used
10. Finish carving	10. Carver, burnishers
11. Remove dental dam (if used)	11. Clamp forceps, scissors
12. Check occlusion	12. Articulating paper and forceps
13. Rinse and evacuate, wipe off markings	13. 2×2 gauze
14. Give posttreatment instructions (pg. 128–129)	
15. Dismiss patient	
16. Perform postprocedure asepsis (pg. 19–20)	

Cavity Preparation and Composite Restoration

Step-by-step procedure	Instruments and materials used
1. Examine oral cavity	1. Basic setup
2. Administer topical and local anesthesia	2. Anesthesia setup
3. Place dental dam (optional)	3. Dental dam setup
4. Remove decay and prepare cavity	4. HP, burs, spoon, hand-cutting instrument
5. Place matrix strip (if Class 2, 3, 4)	5. Mylar matrix strip
6. Rinse, dry, and condition preparation	6. Etchant, applicator
7. Bond and cure	7. Bonding material, applicator, curing light
8. Place composite	8. Composite material and dispenser

Step-by-step procedure	Instruments and materials used
9. Shape composite and cure	9. Composite instrument, curing light
10. Finish and polish composite	10. Sand strips/discs, burs, polishing points
11. Remove dental dam (if used)	11. Clamp forceps, scissors
12. Check occlusion	12. Articulating paper and forceps
13. Rinse and evacuate, wipe off markings	13. 2×2 gauze
14. Give posttreatment instructions (pg. 128–129)	
15. Dismiss patient	
16. Perform postprocedure asepsis (pg. 19–20)	

Crown and Bridge Preparation

Step-by-step procedure	Instruments and materials used
1. Examine oral cavity	1. Basic setup
2. Administer topical and local anesthesia	2. Anesthesia setup
3. Take alginate impression of teeth to be prepared (used for making provisional bridges and crowns)	3. Impression tray, alginate, mixing bowl, and spatula
4. Choose shade	4. Shade guide
5. Prepare crown or bridge abutment	5. High-speed handpiece, diamonds
6. Place retraction material	6. Retraction cord and cord packer
7. Take impression of prepared teeth (if not using triple tray will need bite registration and opposing impression)	7. Impression syringe, tray, and elastomeric impression material

Step-by-step procedure	Instruments and materials used
8. Fabricate temporary crown	8. Temporary material or prefabricated crown
9. Cement temporary crown	9. Temporary luting cement
10. Remove excess cement	10. Scaler, explorer, floss
11. Check occlusion	11. Articulating paper and forceps
12. Rinse and evacuate, wipe off markings	12. 2 × 2 gauze
13. Give posttreatment instructions (pg. 128–129)	
14. Perform postprocedure asepsis (pg. 19–20)	

Crown and Bridge Cementation/Bonding

Step-by-step procedure	Instruments and materials used
1. Examine oral cavity	1. Basic setup
2. Administer local anesthesia if required	2. Anesthesia setup
3. Remove temporary crown	3. Crown remover, hemostat
4. Remove cement	4. Scaler
5. Try-in crown/bridge	5. Floss, articulating paper
6. Adjust fit	6. Diamonds, burs, stones, polishing points
7. Check occlusion	7. Articulating paper and forceps
8. Adjust occlusion as needed	8. Diamonds, burs, stones, and polishing points
9. Clean preparation(s)	9. 2 × 2 gauze, air/water syringe

Step-by-step procedure	Instruments and materials used
10. Cement crown	10. Permanent cement, spatula, mixing pad, plastic instrument, and bite stick
11. Remove excess cement	11. Scaler, floss
12. Rinse and evacuate, wipe off markings	12. 2 × 2 gauze
13. Give posttreatment instructions (pg. 128–129)	
14. Dismiss patient	
15. Perform postprocedure asepsis (pg. 19–20)	

Root Canal

Step-by-step procedure	Instruments and materials used
1. Examine oral cavity	1. Mirror and explorer
2. Administer topical and local anesthesia	2. Anesthesia setup
3. Place dental dam (isolate only one tooth)	3. Dental dam setup
4. Access pulp chamber	4. Handpieces and burs, endo spoon
5. Locate canals	5. Endodontic explorer
6. Remove pulp	6. Broach, files
7. Determine canal(s) length	7. File, stop, file gauge, x-ray
8. Enlarge and shape canals	8. Files (hand and/or rotary), RC Prep

Step-by-step procedure	Instruments and materials used
9. Irrigate and dry canals	9. Sodium hypochlorite, saline, paper points
10. Fit master point	10. Gutta percha, x-ray
11. Cement and condense master point	11. Canal sealer, paste filler, spreader/plugger
12. Cement and condense accessory points	12. Canal sealer, spreader/plugger
13. Sear off the extra gutta percha	13. Heat source, plastic instrument
14. Take final radiograph	
15. Place restoration	

Step-by-step procedure	Instruments and materials used
1. Examine oral cavity	1. Mouth mirror
2. Administer topical and local anesthesia	2. Anesthesia setup
3. Detach periosteum	3. Periosteal elevator
4. Luxate tooth	4. Straight and angular elevators
5. Extract tooth	5. Forceps for specific tooth
6. Curette socket	6. Surgical curette
7. Place gauze	
8. Give posttreatment instructions (pg. 128–129)	
9. Dismiss patient	
10. Perform postprocedure asepsis (pg. 19–20)	

Multiple Extractions and Alveoplasty/Gingivoplasty

Step-by-step procedure	Instruments and materials used
1. Examine oral cavity	1. Mouth mirror
2. Administer topical and local anesthesia	2. Anesthesia setup
3. Make gingival incision	3. Scalpel with #11, #12, or #15 blade
4. Detach periosteum	4. Periosteal elevator
5. Luxate teeth	5. Straight and angular elevators
6. Extract teeth	6. Forceps for specific teeth
7. Curette sockets	7. Surgical curette
8. Remove excess alveolar bone	8. Rongeur and bone file
9. Remove excess gingiva	9. Dean or iris scissors

Step-by-step procedure	Instruments and materials used
10. Irrigate surgical site	10. Irrigating syringe and sterile saline
11. Place sutures	11. Needle holder, sutures, scissors
12. Place gauze	
13. Give posttreatment instructions (pg. 128–129)	
14. Dismiss patient	
15. Perform postprocedure asepsis (pg. 19–20)	

Impacted Tooth Extraction

Step-by-step procedure	Instruments and materials used	Step-by-step procedure	Instruments and materials used
1. Examine oral cavity	1. Mouth mirror	10. Irrigate surgical site	10. Irrigating syringe and sterile saline
2. Administer topical and local anesthesia	2. Anesthesia setup	11. Place sutures	11. Needle holder, sutures, scissors
3. Make gingival incision	3. Scalpel with #11, #12, or #15 blade	12. Place gauze	
4. Detach periosteum	4. Periosteal elevator	13. Give posttreatment instructions (pg.128-129)	
5. Remove bone and/or section tooth	5. Handpiece and burs	14. Dismiss patient	
6. Luxate teeth	6. Straight and angular elevators	15. Perform postprocedure asepsis (pg.19-20)	
7. Extract teeth	7. Forceps or elevators		
8. Remove root fragments, curette socket	8. Root picks, surgical curette		
9. Smooth alveolar bone	9. Rongeur and bone file		

Extraction Forceps

TABLE 12-1

Forceps number	Used for
101	Primary teeth and mandibular permanent incisors
103, 151	Mandibular incisors, canines, and premolars
15, 16, 17, 23	Mandibular molars
222	Mandibular 3rd molars
69	All overlapping anteriors and roots
65	Maxillary overlapping anteriors and roots
99	Maxillary incisors and canines
150	Maxillary incisors, canines, and premolars
18L, 53L, 88L	Maxillary left 1st and 2nd molars
18R, 53R, 88R	Maxillary right 1st and 2nd molars
210	Maxillary 3rd molars

Extraction Forceps Number and Use Illustration

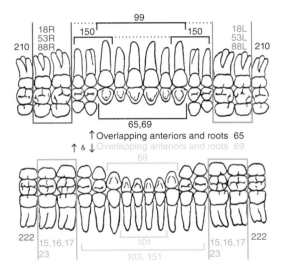

Clinical
Procedures
12

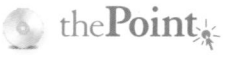

CD-ROM includes extraction forceps review activity.

Posttreatment Instructions

For All Procedures

■ If anesthesia was administered, caution patient to avoid hot beverages and avoid eating until numbness has worn off to prevent damage to soft tissues.

For Restorative Procedures

■ Caution patient to avoid chewing on treated tooth for a few hours.

For Surgical Procedures, Instruct Patient to Do the Following

- Begin pain medication before anesthesia wears off.
- Use ice pack—20 minutes on/20 minutes off—for first 12 to 24 hours to control swelling, after that moist heat can be used.
- Keep gauze pack in for 20 to 30 minutes, replace as needed.
- Avoid vigorous exercise for first 48 hours.
- Avoid smoking, alcohol, and hard foods.
- Do not rinse on the day of surgery, after that rinse three to four times a day with warm salt water.
- Do not suck through a straw or spit.
- Continue brushing and flossing nonsurgical areas.

Notes

Tray Setups

Tray setups include the following:

Restorative Dentistry—Cavity preparation and amalgam restoration, cavity preparation and composite restoration

Fixed Prosthodontics—Crown and bridge preparation, crown and bridge cementation/bonding

Removable Prosthodontics—Denture delivery

Endodontics—Root canal

Periodontics—Prophylaxis, periodontal debridement

Oral and Maxillofacial Surgery—Basic extraction, multiple extraction/alveoplasty/gingivectomy, impaction

Orthodontics—Band seating and bracket bonding, archwire adjustment and tie-in

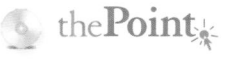

The CD-ROM includes activities and review for the tray setups in this chapter.

Cavity Preparation and Amalgam Tray Setup

Purpose

To provide instrumentation for removing decay and shaping a cavity to hold a restorative material. This material is contoured to restore normal anatomical form.

1. Basic setup
2. Local anesthesia setup
3. Tofflemire matrix band, retainer, and wedges
4. Amalgam well
5. Amalgam capsule
6. Cavity preparation burs
7. Spoon excavator
8. Bin-angle chisel and enamel hatchet (preference of dentist)
9. Amalgam carrier
10. Amalgam condenser
11. Hollenback carver

12. Discoid/cleoid
13. Ball burnisher
14. Hemostat
15. Articulating paper forceps
16. Handpieces (high and low speed)
17. Cavity base/liner
18. Mixing pad and instrument

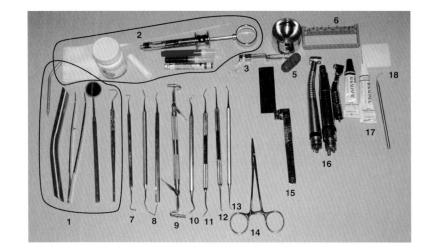

Cavity Preparation and Composite Tray Setup

Purpose

To provide instrumentation for removing decay and shaping a cavity to hold a restorative material. This material is contoured to restore normal anatomical form.

1. Basic setup
2. Local anesthesia setup
3. Cavity preparation burs
4. Spoon excavator
5. Bin-angle chisel and enamel hatchet (preference of dentist)
6. Composite placement instrument
7. Applicator for bonding agent
8. Acid etch
9. Plastic matrix band
10. Bonding agent and disposable well
11. Articulating paper forceps
12. Abrasive strip
13. Abrasive discs and polishing points
14. Handpieces (high and slow speed)
15. Composite compule and dispensing gun

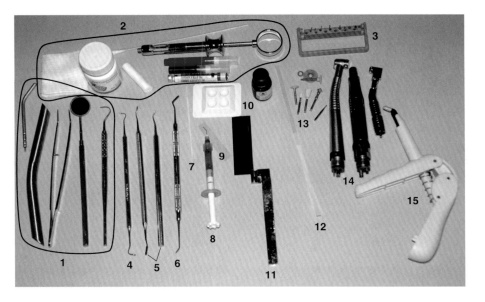

Crown and Bridge Preparation Tray Setup

Purpose

To provide instrumentation for preparing the tooth to support and retain an artificial crown, for making an impression of the tooth preparation, and for fabricating temporary coverage for the prepared tooth.

1. Basic setup
2. Local anesthesia setup
3. Retraction cord
4. Floss
5. Diamonds and burs
6. Handpieces (high and low speed)
7. Spoon excavator
8. Cord packing instrument
9. Plastic instrument
10. Scaler
11. Crown and collar scissors
12. Articulating paper forceps
13. Temporary crowns
14. Contouring pliers
15. Mixing pad
16. Impression material
17. Impression tray
18. Impression paste spatula
19. Impression paste syringe
20. Temporary cement

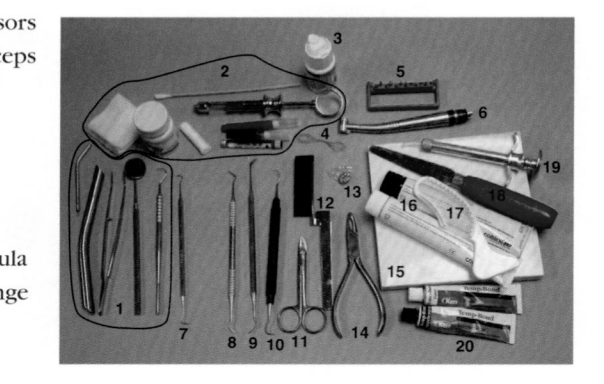

Purpose

To provide instrumentation for removing the temporary coverage, adjusting fit and occlusion of permanent crown or bridge, and permanently cementing or bonding the restoration to the prepared tooth/teeth.

1. Basic setup
2. Local anesthesia setup
3. Crown remover
4. Towel clamp
5. Floss
6. Diamonds and burs
7. Handpieces (high and low speed)
8. Spoon excavator
9. Plastic instrument
10. Scaler
11. Bite stick
12. Articulating paper forceps
13. Cement spatula
14. Permanent cement
15. Mixing pad

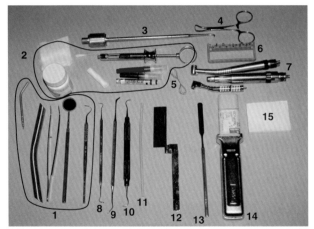

137

Denture Delivery Tray Setup

Purpose

To provide instrumentation for inserting and adjusting the fit and occlusion of a removable denture.

1. Lab burs and stones
2. Pressure indicating paste and cotton applicator
3. Slow-speed handpiece
4. Denture brush
5. A/W syringe tip
6. Mouth mirror
7. Cotton pliers
8. Articulating paper
9. Dentures
10. Hand mirror
11. Dental lathe, sterile rag wheel, and pumice

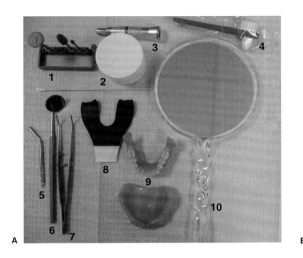

A

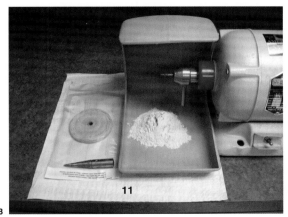

B

Root Canal Tray Setup

Purpose

To provide instrumentation for removing diseased pulp tissue, cleaning and shaping the canal(s), and filling and sealing the canal(s).

1. Dental dam setup
2. Local anesthesia setup
3. File gauge
4. Files
5. Stops
6. Burs
7. Intracanal medications
8. Temporary filling material
9. Air/water syringe tip
10. Oral evacuator tip
11. Cotton pliers
12. Endo explorer
13. Endo excavator
14. Endo spreader
15. Endo plugger
16. Endo plastic instrument
17. Irrigating syringe
18. Irrigating solution
19. Paper points
20. Gutta percha points
21. Handpieces (high and low speed)

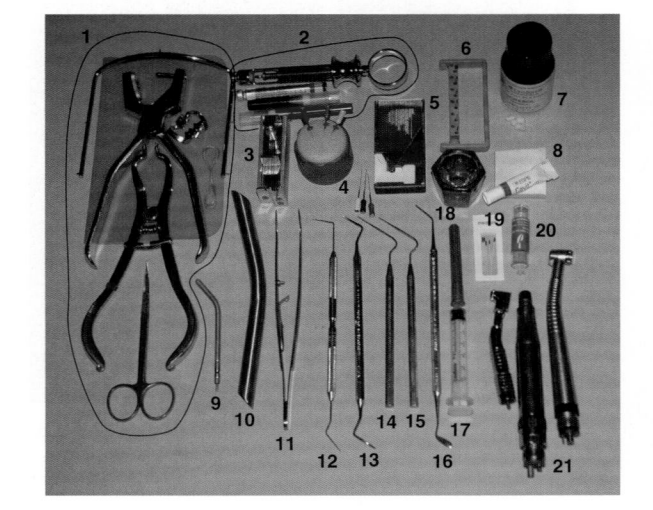

Purpose

To provide instrumentation for removing plaque and calculus from tooth surfaces.

1. Mouth mirror
2. 5 explorer (combination of #23 and #17)
3. 11/12 explorer
4. Periodontal probe
5. Cotton pliers
6. H6/H7 scaler
7. 204S scaler
8. Prophy handpiece
9. Disposable prophy angle with brush
10. Disposable prophy angle with cup
11. Prophy paste
12. Air/water syringe tip
13. Saliva ejector tip
14. Floss
15. 2 × 2 gauze

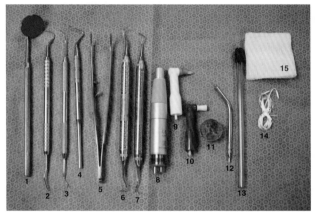

141

Periodontal Debridement Tray Setup

Purpose

To provide instrumentation for removing residual calculus and bacterial toxins from the root surface and gingival wall to promote health and reattachment of the periodontal tissues.

1. Local anesthesia setup
2. Cotton pliers
3. Sharpening stone
4. Mouth mirror
5. 5 explorer (combination of #23 and #17)
6. 11/12 explorer
7. Periodontal probe
8. 204S scaler
9. H6/H7 scaler
10. Gracey curette 1/2
11. Gracey curette 7/8
12. Gracey curette 11/12
13. Gracey curette 13/14
14. Gracey curette 15/16
15. McCalls curette 17/18
16. Air/water syringe tip
17. Oral evacuator tip

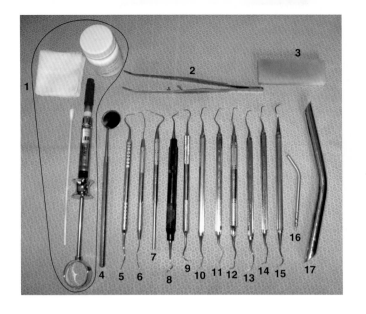

Basic Extraction Tray Setup

Purpose

To provide instrumentation for surgical removal of tooth/teeth.

1. Local anesthesia syringe, needles, and cartridges
2. Sterile gauze
3. Surgical aspirating tip
4. Cotton pliers
5. Mouth mirror
6. Periosteal elevator
7. Straight elevators
8. Surgical curette
9. Hemostat
10. Extraction forceps (selected for specific tooth/teeth)

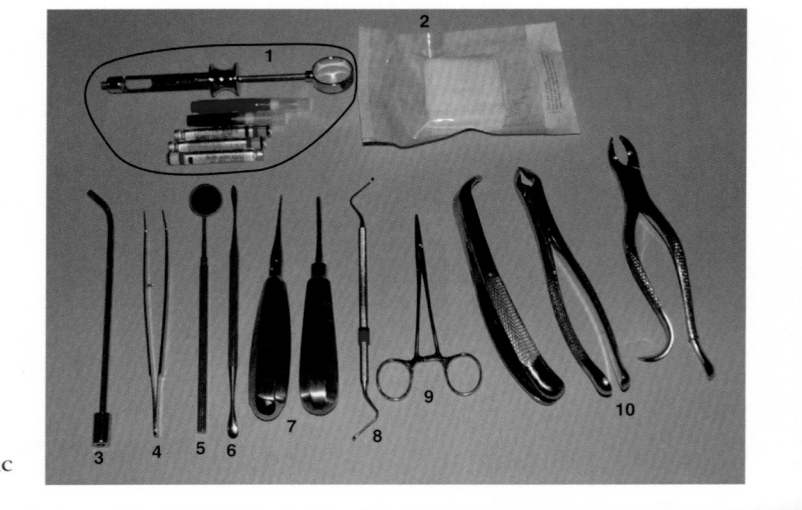

Purpose

To provide instrumentation for surgically removing multiple teeth, reshaping bone and gingiva, and placing sutures.

1. Local anesthesia setup
2. Tissue retractor
3. Scalpel(s)
4. Mouth prop
5. Sterile gauze
6. Surgical aspirating tip
7. Cotton pliers
8. Mouth mirror
9. Periosteal elevator
10. Straight elevators
11. Tissue retractor
12. Surgical curette
13. Bone file
14. Extraction forceps (selected for specific tooth/teeth)
15. Rongeur
16. Tissue scissor
17. Needle holder
18. Hemostat
19. Suture

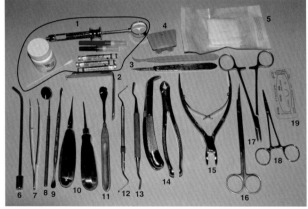

145

Tray
Set-ups
13

Impaction Tray Setup

Purpose

To provide instrumentation for surgically removing impacted tooth. Often involves incision and bone removal.

1. Anesthetic syringe, needles, and cartridges
2. Mouth prop
3. Tissue retractor
4. Austin tissue retractor
5. Surgical bur
6. Hemostat
7. Surgical aspirating tip
8. Mouth mirror
9. Cotton pliers
10. Periosteal elevator
11. Straight elevator
12. Crane pick
13. Angular elevators
14. Root tip picks
15. Surgical curette
16. Molt curette
17. Bone file
18. Tissue scissor
19. Extraction forceps
20. Needle holder
21. Scalpel(s)
22. Suture

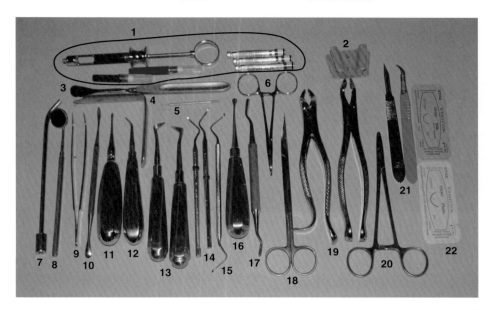

Band Seating and Bracket Bonding Tray Setup

Purpose

To provide instrumentation to fit, position, cement/bond bands and brackets, and tie-in the initial archwire.

1. Brackets and bands on organizer
2. Cement guard
3. Boone positioning gauge
4. Archwire
5. Elastic ligatures
6. Floss
7. Mouth mirror
8. Explorer
9. Cotton pliers
10. Band pusher
11. Band seater
12. Band removing pliers
13. Weingart utility pliers
14. Wire bending pliers
15. Wire cutter
16. Mathieu pliers
17. Distal end cutter
18. Air/water syringe tip
19. Saliva ejector tip

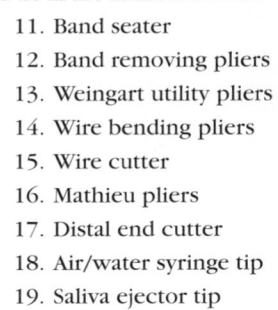

Purpose

To provide instrumentation for archwire adjustment or replacement at periodic intervals.

1. Archwire
2. Elastic ligatures
3. Floss
4. Mouth mirror
5. Explorer
6. Cotton pliers
7. Scaler
8. Weingart utility pliers
9. Wire bending pliers
10. Wire cutter
11. Mathieu pliers
12. Distal end cutter
13. Air/water syringe tip
14. Saliva ejector tip

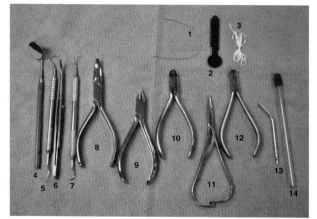

149

Tray
Set-ups
13

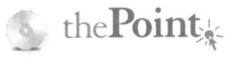 the**Point**

CD-ROM includes additional tray setups: apicoectomy, gingivectomy/gingivoplasty, osteoplasty, suture removal, placing elastic separators, and debanding/debonding.

Clinical Procedures— Expanded Functions

Fabricating a Provisional (Temporary) Crown

Purpose

Provides coverage of prepared teeth to protect from oral fluids and temperature changes and to provide occlusal form and esthetics until the patient returns for laboratory-fabricated crown or bridge.

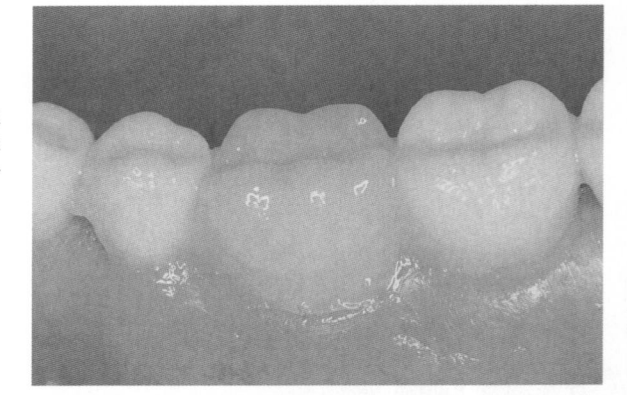

FIGURE 14–1 Provisional crown. Reprinted with permission from Gladwin MA, Bagby M. *Clinical Aspects of Dental Materials: Theory, Practice, and Cases*. 3rd ed. Baltimore, MD: Lippincott Williams & Wilkins; 2008.

Instruments and Materials Needed

Alginate impression or vacuum-formed matrix, provisional crown and bridge material (supplied in cartridge gun and mixing tip), separating medium, ethyl alcohol, cotton pliers, mouth mirror, explorer, scaler, plastic instrument, temporary cement, articulating paper, burs, and finishing discs (Figure 14-2).

Step-by-Step Procedure

1. Before preparation of teeth for crown, take an alginate impression. This will be used as the matrix for the provisional crown or a vacuum-formed matrix can be made.
2. After tooth preparation, dry and lightly lubricate prepared tooth/teeth and surrounding tissue with separating medium (KY jelly, petroleum jelly, or glycerine).
3. Place mixing tip on cartridge gun per manufacturer's directions.
4. Dispense resin into impression/matrix. Start on occlusal surface of tooth that was prepared for crown and then fill to gingival margin.

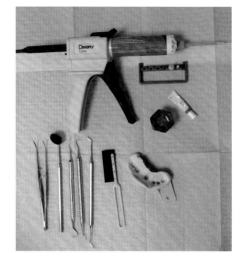

FIGURE 14–2 Provisional crown tray setup.

5. Place impression/matrix over prepared tooth.

6. When the material becomes rubbery (2 to 3 minutes), carefully remove matrix. If restoration remains on tooth, gently remove with cotton pliers or hemostat.

7. Allow to set completely (4 to 5 minutes). Remove oxygen inhibition layer from surface of provisional crown with ethyl alcohol.

8. Remove any excess material; shape and smooth provisional with burs and finishing discs.

9. Place on prepared tooth to check fit.

10. Prepare temporary cement, place in provisional crown, and seat over prepared tooth.

11. Remove excess cement.

12. Check occlusion.

Purpose

To fill and seal pit and fissure grooves on the occlusal surfaces of newly erupted permanent molars to prevent decay.

Instruments and Materials Needed

Basic setup, prophy angle with brush, non-fluoride prophy paste or pumice, cotton rolls and dri-angles or dental dam setup, etch, sealant material, curing light, and articulating paper (Figures 14-4 and 14-5).

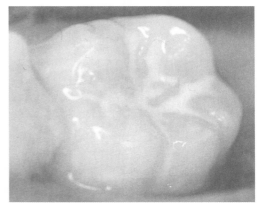

FIGURE 14–3 Dental sealant. Reprinted with permission from Gladwin MA, Bagby M. *Clinical Aspects of Dental Materials: Theory, Practice, and Cases.* 3rd ed. Baltimore, MD: Lippincott Williams & Wilkins; 2008.

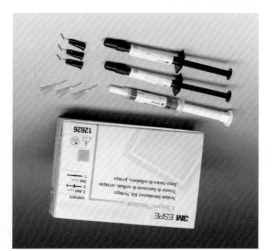

FIGURE 14–5 3M ESPE Clinpro sealant.
Image courtesy of 3M ESPE.

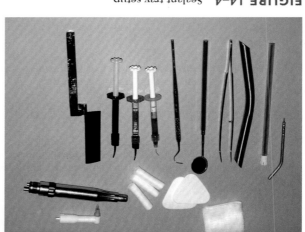

FIGURE 14–4 Sealant tray setup.

Step-by-Step Procedure

1. Thoroughly clean enamel surfaces to be sealed.
2. Isolate and dry teeth.
3. Apply etch to enamel surfaces to be sealed (15 to 60 seconds per manufacturer's instructions).
4. Rinse thoroughly and dry. Verify "frosty" appearance of etched enamel. Repeat if not "frosty" or if etched surfaces come in contact with saliva.
5. Place sealant. Use a stirring or scrubbing motion to apply sealant to pits and fissures with syringe tip, brush, or explorer. Do not overfill.
6. Light cure the sealant.
7. Evaluate for complete coverage and voids.
8. Check occlusion; adjust as necessary.

Coronal Polishing

Purpose

Removal of plaque and stain from tooth surfaces.

Instruments and Materials Needed

Basic setup, prophy handpiece, prophy angle with cup, prophy angle with brush, prophy paste, and floss (Figure 14-6).

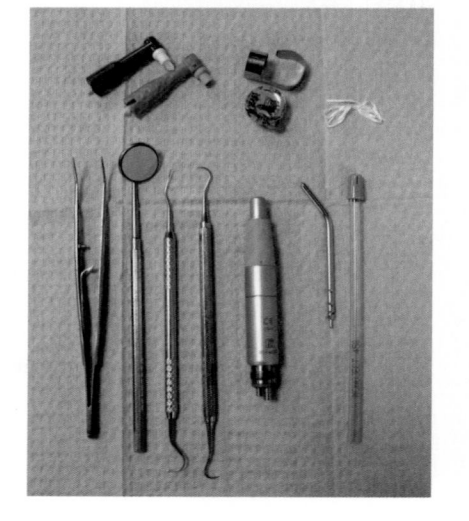

FIGURE 14–6 Coronal polishing tray setup.

Step-by-Step Procedure

1. Explain procedure to the patient.
2. Place prophy angle with cup on handpiece.
3. Pick up polishing paste on rubber cup and place paste on surfaces of two to three of the most posterior teeth in a quadrant.
4. Beginning with the distal surface of the most posterior tooth in a quadrant, adapt the cup to the tooth surface and establish a fulcrum. Keep the fulcrum close to the treatment area, preferably within the same arch.
5. Use slow speed and move the rotating cup with light, patting and wiping strokes.
6. Use only enough pressure to flare the cup slightly. Polish only for a few seconds on each tooth surface.
7. Continue polishing with overlapping strokes. A routine sequence is necessary to prevent missing any teeth. Generally, a quadrant or sextant is polished on the facial and lingual surfaces before moving on to the next area.
8. Use the mouth mirror for retraction and indirect vision as needed.
9. Replenish paste every two to three teeth throughout the procedure.
10. Rinse and evacuate as necessary to maintain patient comfort.

11. After polishing all facial and lingual surfaces, use the prophy brush on the occlusal surfaces.
12. Floss all proximal surfaces.
13. Rinse and evacuate all quadrants.
14. Provide oral hygiene instructions.

Index

Note: The letters 'f' and 't' following the locators refer to figures and tables respectively.